TRANSPLANT: A MEMOIR

More Praise for *Transplant*

"African Americans represent 13% of the US population but account for nearly 35% of people with kidney failure in the US. Bernardine Watson's account of living with a rare kidney disease depicts just how real these statistics are. It is vital that patient advocacy organizations like NephCure and patients like Watson continue to raise awareness and fight for more innovation in the kidney disease space."

—*Kelly Helm, Executive Director of Patient Engagement at NephCure*

"Bernardine Watson has written a beautiful memoir about the struggle to maintain health while living with a potentially lethal disease. But *Transplant: A Memoir* is mostly a book about becoming: a woman, a mother, a member of a family she learns to love better, and a loved and treasured soul mate. Through her struggle, she becomes much more than her disease and bigger and braver than she could have imagined."

—*Marita Golden, Author, Creative Writing Coach, Literary Consultant*

"With honesty and humor, Bernardine Watson takes us on her personal journey to conquer kidney disease, a health condition disproportionately affecting Black people and other people of color in the US. *Transplant: A Memoir,* is also an adult love story, celebrating the power of care and kindness in building a strong relationship."

—*Louis Massiah, Documentary Filmmaker, Founder/Director of Scribe Video Center, Martin Luther King, Jr. Scholar at Massachusetts Institute of Technology*

TRANSPLANT: A MEMOIR

Bernardine Watson

Washington Writers' Publishing House
Washington, DC

Copyright © 2023 by Bernardine Watson

All rights reserved, including the right to reproduce this book or portions thereof in any form whatsoever without written permission except in the case of brief quotations embodied in critical articles or reviews.

COVER DESIGN by Andrew Sargas Klein
BOOK DESIGN and TYPOGRAPHY by Barbara Shaw

ISBN 978-1-941551-36-3

Library of Congress Control Number: 2023940459

Printed in the United States of America

WASHINGTON WRITERS' PUBLISHING HOUSE
2814 5th Street, NE, #1301
Washington, D.C. 20017
More information: www.washingtonwriters.org

In Memory of T, Clint, and Cassandra—
healers in their own ways.

CONTENTS

Acknowledgements viii
Prologue: That Smell 1
1. My Secret Life 6
2. Your Creatinine Level is Creeping Up 38
3. May Day! May Day! 55
4. Everything's Going to be Okay 73
5. Happy New Year to Me 90
6. Me and Baby Alice 100
7. Get Yourself Together 123
8. Happiness is a Man Called Joe 134
9. Traveling and Other Mercies 163
10. Deep in the Belly of the Beast 183
11. An Education 216
12. Time to Make a Move 235
13. Hope! 259
14. Hoping and Waiting 281
15. Loss, Love, Life 305
Epilogue: Fall 2022 312
Book Club Discussion Guide 325

ACKNOWLEDGEMENTS

This book took its time being born, and I want to acknowledge and thank those who helped bring it into the world:

My parents, Alice and Bernard; and my siblings, Alice—my first kidney donor, Judith, Linda, and brother—Bernard Jr, whom we call Jerry. Thank you for loving me.

Joe Davidson, my sweet husband, from whom I continue to learn, every day, about love and life.

Rob Watson, my son, an inspiration from the day he was born; Hakimu and Jasiri, who have expanded my heart.

Naomi Grace, my granddaughter, who keeps me hopeful about the future.

Judy Payne, my altruistic donor and friend.

Valarie Ashley, who was the first to tell me that my story was a book, and who read every page of the draft.

Marita Golden, my incomparable literary coach, who helped me shape a sprawling manuscript into a meaningful whole.

Marilyn Smith, who worked with me on an earlier version of this book.

Kathleen Novak and Jeanie Shackleton, friends who were with me at the beginning of this sojourn and remain in my corner and my heart.

The doctors and technicians who have cared for me, including Nurse Margaret, David Grant, Michael Rudnick, Edward Kraus, Jack Moore, Robert Montgomery, and my current nephrologist, Judith Veis, with whom I trust my life.

Finally, I want to acknowledge NephCure Kidney International, National Kidney Foundation, National Institutes of Health, and other health-related and advocacy organizations that are working on better treatments for kidney disease and equity in the health care system.

Disclaimer

This book is a memoir. It reflects the author's present recollections of experiences over time. Some names and characteristics have been changed, some events have been compressed, and some dialogue has been recreated.

Prologue:
THAT SMELL

Here I am again. Back where I never thought I'd be, especially not on December 22, 2004, just a few days before Christmas. Am I dreaming? If I'm dreaming, somebody please wake me up.

My husband, Joe, parks the car and walks me as far as the front door of 11 Dupont Circle. He's reluctant to leave but has a work meeting.

"Are you sure you'll be okay?" he asks, reaching for my arm.

I'm not at all sure that I'll be okay. I'm trembling on the inside but trying my hardest to look confident and calm on the outside. I look my husband dead in the eye and lie to him, nodding "yes."

"I'll be all right," I say. "I don't think anything much will happen today… probably just an orientation. Whatever happens, I'll handle it. You go on."

I heard myself say "I'll handle it," a familiar refrain coming from me. I'm used to handling things whether I need help or not and am not yet used to a husband who has my back. Frankly, the longer we stand outside the building, the more I want Joe to go. I want to get this first day over with. But my sweet husband won't leave.

"You know I can come back for you around ten thirty, right? That's the time you'll be finished, right?" he asks, pulling at my coat sleeve for emphasis.

"Baby, I'm pretty sure I'll be able to drive myself home," I say, feigning patience. "You don't have to come back over here. Besides, I don't know exactly how long I'll be. Like I said, today will probably be an orientation. Listen, let me go on in. I don't want to be late."

"All right," Joe says, tugging at my coat sleeve again. "I'll be back for you at ten thirty. You're not driving today. Maybe the next time, but not today. I need to see the inside of this place, anyway. I want to see where my baby will be."

I hug him with one arm and pull at the heavy glass door of the building with the other.

A guard is sitting at the desk in the building's lobby reading the newspaper. Before I can ask him for directions, he glances at me and mumbles, "Dialysis, right? Take the elevator down one to the basement," and returns to reading his paper.

I stand glued to the floor, stunned into immobility. That man has no idea that he's tapped into a deep insecurity of mine and hit me with a very low blow. What is it about me that makes him think I could only be going to the dialysis center? Aren't there at least four more floors and many other offices in this building?

After a few weeks of coming to 11 Dupont Circle, I understand exactly why the guard drew the conclusion he had. Most of the Black people who come into this lobby every day are going down to the basement for dialysis. But on my first day in the building, I have no idea who comes in and out. His assumption pisses me off. *How dare he*, I think as I check my reflection in the elevator mirror. Do I look like a dialysis patient? Is that all I am now? Is it all "down" from here?

The elevator doors open into a dark vestibule, which doesn't seem to belong to the rest of this brightly lit, beautifully landscaped building. As I turn to my right, the first thing I see through the windows of the vestibule doors is a disturbingly large, white banner with big, bold, black and red letters in case I have any doubt about where I am:

FRESENIUS MEDICAL CARE, DUPONT CIRCLE DIALYSIS CENTER

The waiting area on the other side of the doors is lined with rows of plastic folding chairs. All the chairs I can see are filled with Black people talking, laughing, and drinking coffee or soda. Some are eating what look like breakfast sandwiches from fast-food restaurants. Ugh. I stand for a while outside the doors looking in. The scene looks like a group of people at a social gathering rather than patients waiting to be hooked up to machines.

"How the hell am I going to do this?" I ask myself under my breath. "These are not my people." I have no choice, and I enter.

Oh my god, that smell. An awful but familiar odor hits me in the face as soon as I enter the room. I place my hand over my nose and mouth to keep from inhaling the putrid air. Immediately, I am flooded with memories of my first go-round with dialysis—a brief two-month stint before my first transplant in 2000, at Philadelphia's Presbyterian Hospital. The center at that hospital smelled as foul as this one. A dialysis technician at the Presbyterian center told me that the stench came from the chemicals used to clean the dialysis machines. I had no reason to doubt the guy, but to me, the odor seems a more sinister mixture of blood, sweat, tears, fear, human body waste, and yes, death.

Looking for a place to sit down and steady myself, I grab the first empty chair. With my head lowered, eyes squeezed shut, and coat still wrapped tightly around my body, I hope no one will bother me. I need a moment to get myself together. I can't seem to calm my racing mind and pounding heart. I can hear a yoga teacher telling me to "breathe" and "be in the moment." But I don't want to breathe this air, and the present moment, in this chair, in this room, in this building, is the very last place I want to be. Swaddled in my cocoon, I retreat to the narrative that has been playing in my head since my kidney failure the week before.

I shouldn't be here. I shouldn't be facing dialysis again. Everyone—all the doctors and nurses who treated me before, during, and after my transplant—were so certain I'd be okay. My older sister, Alice, had been my donor, which almost guaranteed a successful transplant. I remember the transplant doctor at the University of Pennsylvania Hospital, where the surgery took place, saying confidently, "You and your sister are a perfect blood and tissue match. You should do very well. This transplant should last you at least twenty years." I believed them. My family had prayed for me incessantly. Where did those prayers go? Was all that praying for naught? I'd fallen woefully short of "doing very well." After not quite five years, I am sitting in the lobby of Fresenius Medical Care, once again waiting for my turn at the dialysis machine. Merry Christmas to me.

I'd counted on the doctors to be right. I have plans—a life to live, milestones to achieve. As far as I was concerned, I'd been a bit of a late bloomer and needed to make up for lost time. A few missteps in my youth had landed me behind my peers on the professional development curve. At age nineteen, instead of experiencing life on a college campus, I was married with a baby.

For several years I'd lived on welfare and food stamps and dragged my baby boy through more ratty living situations than I want to remember while I scratched and clawed my way through college.

In 1984, at thirty-three years old, and with a great new job and two dysfunctional marriages behind me, I thought I was poised to fly. However, that year, for reasons I will never understand, I was diagnosed with a kidney disease that had a name I couldn't pronounce—Focal Segmental Glomerulosclerosis (FSGS). According to the doctor who gave me the horrible news, FSGS had the potential to destroy my kidneys and kill me. Did I fall apart? No. I handled it. I pulled myself together like the tough South Philly girl I am and spent the next fifteen years working and striving to stay as healthy as I could, telling almost no one about my condition. Why should I? My diagnosis was nobody's business but mine. Besides, who wants the pity or curiosity of sympathizers? I certainly didn't.

FSGS was my secret until I couldn't keep the secret anymore. By 1999, the year my daddy died, my diminishing kidney function began to make me ill. I'll never forget the day a nephrologist told me, "You're going to need dialysis or a kidney transplant soon."

The doctor was right. I needed both. I went through all that back in 2000. Now here I am again.

Chapter One:
MY SECRET LIFE

In 1984, when I was thirty-three years old, living in the Twin Cities, and newly separated from my second husband, my gynecologist found protein in my urine during a routine examination. She suggested that I see a nephrologist. My friend Kathleen, who went with me to the appointment, remembers the gynecologist saying that my condition could be serious. I'd already been through a lot in my life—poverty, welfare, teen pregnancy, and two disastrous marriages—so I didn't let her concern worry me very much. Besides, I hadn't heard anything about kidney disease running in my family. Don't get me wrong, there is plenty of illness on both my mother's and father's sides. Diabetes? Both my father and his father before him had "sugar," as many in my community call the disease. In fact, the one time I met my father's father, he was sitting in a wheelchair with both legs amputated from the ravages of diabetes. High blood pressure? Show me a Black family with no high blood pressure. As a kid, eavesdropping on grown folks' conversations, I heard my older relatives complain about their "pressure" all the time. Alcoholism and drug addiction? While fortunately, neither of my parents suffered these afflictions, plenty of people on both sides of my extended family did. But kidney disease? At the time I was diagnosed, I'd never heard anyone in the family mention it.

Despite my attitude, I decided to follow my gynecologist's recommendation and consult a kidney specialist. This young gynecologist had come highly recommended by several female acquaintances, and she'd taken good care of me during my years in the Twin Cities. Besides, I had a good job and good health insurance. Seeing the specialist couldn't hurt. I was certain that the protein in my urine was a fluke, or an anomaly caused by the stress of my failing marriage.

My friend Jeanie insisted on going with me to the biopsy procedure. I felt perfectly capable of going alone, but Jeanie wouldn't hear of it. She was one of the few close friends I'd made in Minneapolis and one of the only people I'd told my secret. We'd met at Control Data Corporation, the Minneapolis computer company where we both worked, and immediately bonded over our love of fashion and soul music. We also had something even more significant in common—we were single mothers of sons, which bound us even more closely. Jeanie is White, but she's as brown in coloring as many of the Black women I know, and just as soulful. She's also tiny but seasoned by more than her fair share of tough breaks in life. I respected, loved, and trusted her enough to let her see me vulnerable.

The nephrologist wasn't crazy about Jeanie being in the procedure room but finally gave in to my repeated requests. Jeanie stood beside the operating table wearing a gown and mask, holding my hand, and watching as the doctor guided a needle into my back and pulled out a small piece of my kidney tissue. Pointing to pictures of my kidneys projected onto a screen, the doctor explained that I had a relatively rare disease of the kidney called FSGS, short for Focal Segmental Glomerulosclerosis. For many people like me, he explained, there is no known cause for FSGS. The disease attacks the kidney's filtering units, called glomeruli, and causes serious scarring, which allows too much protein to be released into the urine. According to this nephrologist, FSGS could lead to permanent kidney damage and even failure. He pointed to highlighted sections of my kidneys and asked, "Can you see the scarring, Ms. Watson? The damage is minimal at this point, but it's real."

Honestly, I couldn't tell which portions of my kidneys were scarred. All I could see were two bean-shaped globs of red flesh on either side of my spine. If my kidneys were diseased, I'd have to take the doctor's word for it. I was too stunned to see much of anything. I looked over at Jeanie who was squeezing my hand tightly. She shook her head reassuringly as if to tell me that things would be okay. But all I could think was *FSGS? What the hell? How can I possibly have a life-threatening disease? I'm only thirty-three years old!*

The doctor waited patiently as I stared blankly at the pictures of my insides. Eventually, as we sat in his office, he patted my arm and said sympathetically,

"Ms. Watson, I know this is a lot for you to take in. However, you've told me that you've been fatigued for some time and your gynecologist sent you to me because of the protein in your urine. Both are symptoms of FSGS. Now we have the biopsy results to support that diagnosis. Ms. Watson, FSGS is a serious disease with no known cure. If your FSGS results in kidney failure, the only options will be dialysis or a kidney transplant. You need to be followed regularly."

In the doctor's waiting room, Jeanie put her arms around

me and reluctantly said goodbye. She had to get back to work. The receptionist looked at me expectantly as I passed her desk, but I didn't stop to make a follow-up appointment. I walked out of the office with as much calm and dignity as I could muster. FSGS? I couldn't even pronounce the full name of this disease. As I drove back to my apartment in St. Paul, the sky opened with a violent rainstorm. I started to cry too. Why not? I was in my own car. No one could see or hear me. Out of habit, I pushed the radio dial. The song *96 Tears* by Mark and the Mysterians was playing, and I sobbed along.

That day was a rare moment for me. I wouldn't cry like that again for a long time. Although I'd been living in the Twin Cities for almost three years, I was still a South Philly girl, raised to be tough, and self-reliant. I didn't call my family back in Philly and tell them what was going on with me and I had no intention of telling my twelve-year-old son, Robert. One of the reasons I'd come to the Twin Cities in the first place was to give my son a more carefree childhood than he could have in Philadelphia. I certainly wasn't going to tell him that I had a disease that could kill me.

In addition to Jeanie, I eventually told two more friends, Kim and Kathleen, about the time bomb that could be ticking away inside me. With the breakup of my marriage and now this dreadful health news, even I needed a few friends to help steady me. Finally, I told my estranged husband, Alexs. I owed him money and used my awful diagnosis to buy some time and a little sympathy. I told no one else. As a young girl, I learned well from my family and community that life could be unfair, even mean. There was nothing and almost no one I could truly count on but myself, even if my own body proved unreliable.

I grew up in a Black, poor to working-class neighborhood in South Philly, just blocks away from the 7th Ward area where

BERNARDINE WATSON

W.E.B. DuBois did his landmark, 1899 sociological study, "The Philadelphia Negro." My grandparents, on both sides, came to Philadelphia from Virginia and Florida, as part of the Great Migration, when, according to the DuBois study, between 1910 and 1930, over 1.5 million Black citizens left the Jim Crow South and poured into the north seeking freedom and economic opportunity. Philadelphia was a major destination for Black people fleeing southern oppression. In 1900, the Black population of the city was approximately 63,000. By 1920, a few years before both of my parents' birth, the City's Black population had more than doubled to approximately 134, 000.

My parents, Alice and Bernard, both from large, struggling families, had five children: Alice, named for my mom and often called Baby Alice, Me—Bernardine, but nicknamed B or BB, Judith, Linda, and the youngest and only boy, Bernard Jerome Jr., or Jerry. All seven of us lived in a tiny, rickety, row house at 1437 Montrose Street. Grandma Daisy Hayes, who'd separated from my grandfather, Samuel, when my father was a boy, lived next door. Daddy's sister, Aunt Betty lived down the street with her children, and scores of aunts, uncles, and cousins lived within walking distance.

We were the Hayes clan, well known and respected in the neighborhood as people who didn't bother anyone if no one bothered them. For much of his adult life, Daddy worked on construction sites as a mason tender— an onsite assistant to the stonemason, who helped organize tools, transport materials, and keep the job site clean. My father was a highly intelligent man, who later in life told me how much he hated that job and how disrespectfully he was treated by White co-workers. "I'm fortunate that I didn't kill someone on that job," he admitted. But Daddy got up between four and five every morning and went to work to support his family. In the early 1970s, when my father was in his forties, he got a job as a business agent for Laborer's Local 332 and later proudly served as the local's vice president.

Mommy was a homemaker until my little brother Jerry was old enough for school, then she worked first as a kindergarten aid and later as a clerk-typist for the Philadelphia School District. Grandma Daisy dipped ice cream on weekdays in the basement of John Wanamaker's Department Store. However, to supplement her income, she also ran a speakeasy out of her home on the weekends, selling booze and chicken or fish dinners and renting rooms to customers who "got lucky" or were just too drunk to go home.

With few exceptions, we and the neighbors we lived among were hardworking people. We loved each other, fought each other, and looked out for each other. At the same time, despite our closeness, in proximity and emotion, everyone did what they could to keep their personal business to themselves. In our world, people came and went, babies were born and died, folks coupled and broke up, and fortunes rose and fell without much open discussion of the circumstances.

"Ain't nobody's business" was the unspoken, and when necessary, spoken mantra. My father, Bernard, often told us, "What happens in this house stays here." There would be hell to pay if he ever heard that one of us put family business in the street. Of course, there was always gossip, but engaging in too much idle prattle could be dangerous to your well-being. My Aunt Betty once punched our neighbor, Miss Louise, in the face and sent her to the hospital, for gossiping about some nefarious activity she'd seen going on in my aunt's house.

"She should have stayed out of my business," was the only reason Aunt Betty ever gave for the assault.

When I think back on the people I grew up with, their attitudes about others poking around in their private affairs make sense to me. Most in my family and community didn't have much more than their pride, and they wanted to keep it. Life was hard enough without everyone knowing your ups and downs, offering their two cents about how you ought to live your life, or even worse, using the information to make you feel lower than you already did. This philosophy and way of life, which molded me as a child, influenced the way I lived my life as an adult and faced FSGS.

"You'd better know how to take care of yourself" was another tenet I heard early and often. My father took good care of us as children, but when I came home pregnant at nineteen years old, he made it clear that I had to find another place to live. Bringing "shame" on the family wasn't an option. "If you want to act grown," he told me, "You need to get out of my house." A few weeks later, I did. Likewise, once I understood that I needed to fight for my health, I knew that the fight was up to me and no one else.

∼

EVENTUALLY, I learned to pronounce the name of my disease correctly: fo-cal seg-men-tal glo-mer-u-lo-scle-ro-sis. Also, by reading articles from the National Institutes of Health, National Kidney Foundation, NephCure Kidney International and the Mayo and Cleveland Clinic websites, I learned about its horrible effects. I read that African Americans had approximately four times the risk of FSGS as European Americans. Like most kidney diseases, FSGS damages the kidney and causes waste to build up in the body. Kidney disease generally is so destructive because it can cause other major, deadly health problems such as heart disease and increase the risk of stroke or heart attack. However, FSGS is considered particularly pernicious. Within five to twenty years of onset, the kidney scarring caused by FSGS meant total kidney failure for most patients. The only treatments to try and prevent kidney failure focused on slowing the progression of the disease by using steroids to improve kidney function, medications to keep blood pressure under control, diuretics to help the body get rid of excess fluids, and dietary changes such as reducing salt, to lighten the load on the kidneys. Often these treatments were unsuccessful. Unfortunately, despite FSGS's significant health burden, there were few therapeutic options for those who suffered from the disease and the therapies available often had significant toxic effects on patients. This disease I was dealing with was no joke.

While I was beginning to understand the seriousness of my FSGS diagnosis, I procrastinated in seeking follow-up care. Despite my toughness, I feared the disease. However, I wasn't crazy, and several months after the biopsy, I finally made an appointment for a second opinion with a nephrologist at the Mayo Clinic in Rochester, Minnesota. What was the point of living in Minnesota if I couldn't take advantage of having the best hospital in the world just a few hours from my home? Maybe a doctor at the famed Clinic would look at my biopsy and see something more benign than the dreaded FSGS. Maybe, with Mayo's focus on research and innovation, they could save my kidneys. Maybe, by some miracle, a Mayo Clinic doctor would tell me I'd been misdiagnosed, that I didn't have kidney disease at all, that the whole business had been a medical error.

In June of 1985, I enlisted my friend, Kim, to drive me approximately two hours south on Route 52 from Minneapolis to Rochester. Kim and I met in a women's group and became unlikely comrades. Both of us had joined the group in search of a direction in life, but beyond feeling adrift in the world, we would seem to have nothing else in common. Kim looked like the kind working-class, bleached blond that I might have looked down on, had I passed her in the grocery store. However, once I got to know her, I found that I identified with her gritty determination to overcome an unhappy childhood and make a good life for herself. Besides, she loved Black culture and Black men. After I'd lived in predominately White Minnesota for a few years, her true appreciation of "Blackness" endeared her to me immensely. We had fun together and sometimes I needed to forget my troubles and just have fun.

I was ecstatic when Kim agreed to drive to Rochester with me. I had never been very good with directions and feared I'd get lost and miss my appointment at the Clinic. Further, I needed more than the car radio to keep me company. I was on edge, and left on its own, my mind would begin to race around and around with questions and recriminations: Why is this happening to me? Why didn't I go to the doctor when I first started feeling fatigued? Maybe if I had listened to my body, I wouldn't be in this fix now! Kim, who talked incessantly, was my insurance policy against arriving at the Mayo Clinic a complete basket case.

I didn't know at the time that the doctor I would see that day at Mayo, Dr. James V. Donadio, was a world-famous nephrologist and an emeritus professor at the Clinic's College of Medicine. However, over the years of my sojourn with FSGS, whenever I'd recite my medical history to a new doctor and mentioned Donadio's name, I'd see a spark of true engagement in their eyes.

"You've been examined by Jim Donadio?" they'd ask with surprise. I'd pull out the follow-up letter from Donadio as my ultimate trump card. That letter had magical powers. Suddenly, after viewing Donadio's scrawling signature at the bottom, I'd see doctors perk up and pay a little more attention to me. I could almost read the inner dialogue behind their more attentive eyes. *If this little Black woman is smart enough to get in to see Donadio, maybe she's worth my time.*

Frankly, I don't remember how I got Donadio's name. I'm certain that in making an appointment at the Clinic, I only asked to see a nephrologist, not the most famous doctor in the Mayo Clinic's Division of Nephrology and Hypertension. I also hadn't really expected a miracle from the Mayo Clinic but the news he gave me wasn't all bad. When the follow-up letter from Donadio's office arrived a week or so after my visit, I skipped over the details of my physical examination and the medical gobbledygook about lepocytes and macrocytes, looking for his bottom-line assessment of my condition. Finally, I read these lines near the end of the letter,

"We reviewed the outside renal biopsy… and our kidney pathologist thought that the changes showed mild mesangioproliferative and sclerosing glomerular changes and focal moderate small vessel sclerosis. These changes represent a chronic scarring process, but your normal kidney function and only mild proteinuria show that it is not thus far adversely affecting your kidneys. I think your overall prognosis is quite good."

The letter ended with the same blah, blah, blah I'd already heard before about needing to be followed regularly by a nephrologist. There. I had to accept it. I had FSGS. However, as far as I was concerned, the most important words in the letter were "your prognosis is quite good." I let those five words sink into my mind and body and waited to feel their impact. First came a cool sense of relief that I probably wouldn't face kidney failure or dialysis any time soon or possibly ever. Next came gratitude. First, I was grateful to myself for having sense enough to get a second opinion from one of the best clinics in the world. FSGS was still my reality, but at least now I knew more than the worst possible scenario I'd heard from the first nephrologist. Second, I was grateful to Dr. Donadio for the sliver of hope his optimistic diagnosis provided.

Still, since I'd never been a person who could see the glass as "half full," deep down inside, I believed something had gone terribly wrong inside my body. My prognosis might be "good," but hadn't this disease attacked me out of the blue? What's to stop it from getting worse despite Donadio's forecast? In dark moments, I pummeled myself with doubts and questions. "Why did my body let me down this way? Didn't I lead a healthy life? Wasn't I the only one in the family who watched my diet and exercised regularly? Hadn't I worked hard to get a college education and get myself out of poverty? Didn't everyone say I had a great future?" Now, that future could be in jeopardy because of this damn disease.

FSGS was not supposed to happen to me. Because of my good health habits, I'd been sure that I wouldn't be a candidate for any of the diseases — like heart disease, high blood pressure, diabetes, or yes, kidney disease— that ran rampant through Black communities. I thought I'd left all that behind when I escaped poverty. Now, I felt marked, singled out for a punishment I didn't deserve. Honestly, I felt ashamed for being sick at all. I vowed repeatedly not to tell anyone else about my illness.

"Why should I give anyone this information," I rationalized. So they can feel sorry for me? I had my pride and didn't want anyone's sorrow or pity. Why should I tell my parents and siblings? So they can worry about me? So my mother can have heart failure like she did when she found out I was pregnant at

19? Why should I give this news to my son? To scare him? No. I had a position to play as a strong woman—mother, daughter, and sister. Besides, whatever was going on inside my body was my personal business—no one else's.

While I believe strongly that part of my initial attitude toward the FSGS diagnosis was a direct result of my upbringing, research says that people across race, class, and economic levels often go to great lengths to hide a grim illness. Years later, when I read psychotherapist Katie Willard Virant's analysis of the intersection between illness and shame in our culture, her words hit close to home. In the March 2019 issue of *Psychology Today*, she draws on Susan Sontag's "Illness as Metaphor" to write, "To be ill is to be suspect. What did you do to cause your illness? What aren't you doing to cure it? Illness is not just about the body malfunctioning, it's about the ill person's character. Shame comes from the internalization of this cultural belief that we are somehow at fault for getting ill and continuing to be ill…. When we are ashamed of being ill, we don't talk about our illness to others." I held my secret close.

By 1986, I was ready to leave the Twin Cities. I'd come to the Midwest in 1981 with a new husband and high hopes for giving my ten-year-old son the "good life" in a region that, at the time, topped all the lists of "best places in the country" to live. After five years, however, I'd had enough of the cold, the blonds, the pale faces, and the "Minnesota Nice" attitude. My marriage was "all over but the shoutin'" and the "good job" I'd found at Control Data Corporation (CDC) was probably the next thing to go. In the 1980's CDC was a major computer company located in Bloomington, Minnesota, just outside of Minneapolis. I worked in a section of the company dedicated to selling computers and computer-based learning programs to underserved communities in the U.S. and internationally. I did well at CDC for a while. I even traveled to Jamaica, West Indies, and New Zealand to train educators in how to use CDC's education products. By the mid-1980's however, Control Data had begun to hemorrhage money and rumors abounded that my job, along with those of hundreds more, would be eliminated.

An offer of employment in Philly was almost enough to make me believe in divine intervention. A friend and colleague I worked with in the past had started a small consulting firm. When he needed to expand, he reached across the country to bring me back home. I told him nothing about my illness. After all the tumult I'd experienced in the past few years, I saw this stroke of good fortune as something I deserved. Just maybe, the future still held promise for me.

As I prepared to go back east and my Twin Cities experiment faded into the distance, I reflected on the time I'd spent in the middle of the country. In many ways, the years had been brutal. The weather was more bitter than anything I'd ever experienced. I'd been deprived of the omnipresent Black culture I'd taken for granted on the east coast. My marriage crumbled. Still, I didn't leave the Minneapolis-St. Paul without regrets. I'd made a few friends—women co-workers; members of a Thursday night women's group; White working-class daughters of America's heartland—women I never would have met had I not gone west. Most had come to Minneapolis-St. Paul from places like Hibbing, a small city on Minnesota's iron range, two hundred miles north of the Twin Cities; or farming communities and small towns in surrounding states like North or South Dakota, Iowa, and Wisconsin. Most left home to escape an unhappy family life or what they saw as limited horizons.

I was struck by the experiences I had in common with these women, despite the differences in our backgrounds. One friend told me how her father insisted she attend the local community college after high school and slapped her hard across the face when she argued that she be allowed to attend the University of Minnesota. Her admission shocked me. I thought only poor, Black girls like me got slapped across the face by their fathers. These women were anchors for me during my years in the Twin Cities when I knew few Black people well. One let me stay in her apartment after I left my husband, until I could find my own place. Another stored my furniture in her basement. Kathleen, who was the first to hear that I might have a serious kidney disease, Jeanie, who accompanied me to my first biopsy, and Kim who drove me to the Mayo Clinic, will always be part of my "FSGS" story. However, at the time, I wasn't sure if any of these friendships would survive the distance—literally and figuratively—between the east coast and the Midwest. I thought they might very well fade with time, which made our goodbyes especially poignant.

There was also my ex-husband, Alexs. We'd seen little of each other after our sad separation. When I left our marriage, I put a river between us by moving across the Mississippi to St. Paul, leaving him in the "cute little house" we'd bought together in Minneapolis. I heard scuttlebutt that he moved on with a woman I suspected him of dating before we split. Nevertheless, I couldn't leave the Twin Cities without seeing him. There was a time when Alexs and I were deliriously in love and inseparable. The move to the mid-west had blown up in our faces, but for me, our relationship was much bigger than this bad chapter. He'd always be in my blood, like family. We hardly said a word the day we met to say goodbye. All we could do was put our arms around each other and hold on for a few moments.

As happy as I was to be going home, I knew the circumstances of our return were not perfect. Nothing reminded me of that reality more than the foul smell that hit Robby and me in the face as we crossed the Platt bridge on the way into the city from the airport. Since I was a kid, I'd known the smell of rotten eggs or cabbage cooking that emanated from the refineries outside the airport. I'm sure this smell has contributed to one of the City's nicknames "Filthadelphia." My mom was from Elmwood (also known as Eastwick, Tinicum, or the Meadows.) a semi-rural community that bordered the airport, where Blacks and other ethnic groups had lived together surprisingly peacefully for decades. On just about every Sunday, my father would drive the family out to Elmwood to visit my maternal grandmother, Elizabeth Grace. Going and coming over the "Platt," we were treated to the same scent that some thirty years later still sullied the City's air. "Ah, I'm home," I laughed to myself. "Some things about Philly never change."

But five years is a long time to be away from a city, and a big, complicated place like Philadelphia waits for no one. Lots had happened in Philly since I'd left in 1981, including the election, in 1984 of Wilson Goode, the City's first African American mayor. The next year, that same Mayor ordered explosives dropped on a house in West Philly, occupied by the Black liberation and back to nature organization, MOVE. Eleven people were killed, including five children. Sixty homes were destroyed, and some would say the city's soul was permanently scarred. Some would tell me that if I wasn't in the city for the MOVE incident, I wasn't a true Philadelphian anymore.

Our return to Philadelphia in the summer of 1986 also coincided with a devastating change in many American cities across the country, the arrival of powerfully addictive crack cocaine. The hardest-hit cities were in the Northeast and Mid-Atlantic, including Philadelphia, where, by 1985 a Jamaican "posse" had a vicious presence selling millions of dollars of crack, cocaine, and marijuana from street corners and drug houses in the city's poorest neighborhoods.

I couldn't pretend that I wasn't nervous about bringing Robby back to our hometown now. My son was fifteen and already rebelling against my authority. This behavior started a few years before when he began to openly flout my curfews, hanging out late into the night with friends. I didn't worry about him too much in Minneapolis, where the streets seemed much safer. But Philadelphia was far from Minneapolis.

In addition to my worries about safety, Robby wasn't thrilled about leaving the Twin Cities, where he'd settled in better than I had. He was leaving friends and most important to him at the time, a girlfriend behind. I can't remember the girlfriend's name—Suzy, Tiffany, or something like that. I knew she was blonde, and that alone was enough to make me want to leave town. If my son was going to end up with a White girl, a blonde no less, I wanted it to be because he'd dated an array of girls, including Black girls, and chosen a White one, not because little blonde Barbie dolls were all there were to choose from.

As far as I was concerned, I had no choice but to come back home to Philadelphia. The Twin Cities had pulled the welcome mat out from under me. My marriage was over, and my job was about to disappear. Furthermore, I had no idea what might happen to my health. One doctor told me that my FSGS could cause kidney failure or even death, while the other said my prognosis was "very good." How the hell was I supposed to handle that kind of uncertainty? The only thing I knew how to do was to keep moving forward, and at this point, forward meant going back . . . home to Philly. "If I'm going to be sick," I thought, "I'm better off living closer to family than way out in the Twin Cities where all I had was a few friends." I hadn't been close to my family in years, but they were family. Despite any differences, my family would come if I needed them. Not that I expected to need anyone. Thank goodness I had a job and could take care of myself and my son. Like Billie Holiday sang. "God bless the Child." I'd do the best I could for me and Robby.

Once back home, I left Robby with my parents while I stayed with a friend and looked for a place for us to settle. Mommy was overjoyed to have her grandson staying in her house but was hurt by my choice to go elsewhere.

"I thought you were coming home," she said in her sad voice as we stood in the living room surrounded by graduation pictures of her children and other memorabilia she loved. I recognized the hurt in Mommy's voice and could see the ache in her eyes. While I didn't want to cause Mommy any pain, the truth was that the house where we were standing had never been my home. My parents brought the house, a three-story Georgian Stone structure in the Logan section of Philly, in 1970, a few months after I'd left the family at nineteen-years-old, pregnant, and alone. After living with their five children in a tiny, rented South Philly rowhouse for years, this house was my parents' dream. But it wasn't mine. Once when I was in college and having financial difficulties, my father convinced me to bring Robby and come stay at the family home while I finished school. Robby's and my stay only lasted three months, since like during most of my childhood, Daddy and I couldn't get along. All these years later, I still found it difficult to stay under my parents' roof for very long.

Mommy and I stood staring at each other. The house was quiet. It was Saturday evening and Daddy was probably out playing pinochle with friends he'd known since childhood. Robby had gone up to the third floor of the house to watch television. I knew Mommy understood why I couldn't stay. We both remembered that night in our old house on Montrose Street after I told her and Daddy I was pregnant. In fact, in the few seconds that Mommy and I stood staring at each other, the whole Montrose Street scene played out again in the space between us. As if on a stage set, I saw the kitchen's yellow, grease-stained walls; smelled the fried silver trout we'd eaten for dinner that night and heard the television set blasting from the living room. Just like that night, Daddy raged at me:

"You out here fuckin' around while I'm trying to send you to some school. You out here fuckin' around like every other whore up and down this block? I won't have that in my house."

I was too old for Daddy to beat me with a belt like he'd done when I was younger, but his words fell on me just as hard as the blows I remembered. No matter how many years passed, I'd never gotten over how Daddy treated me that night. While Mommy and I had never talked about that horrible scene, I knew instinctively that she remembered every second just as I did: Me standing frozen in fear and shock at Daddy's attack, my feet stuck to the tattered linoleum floor; my boyfriend Bob bolting for the front door, unable to stand the heat in the kitchen; Mommy tearfully murmuring "No, Bernard, no." We also never talked about what happened next: how I started to bleed from all the stress, Daddy's refusal to take me to the hospital, she and

I going to Philadelphia General on the bus; me leaving home for good the next day.

My body shuddered as I tried unsuccessfully to shake off those old memories. So much had happened in my life since those ugly days. After I left home, I changed my nickname to Dine, putting more than physical distance between me and my family of origin. In the fall of 1970, Bob and I married, and I went to live with his family. About five months later, on January 19, 1971, Robby was born. A few years afterward, Bob and I separated, then divorced. I went on to finish college, remarry and move to Minneapolis, and divorce again.

Now I was back in Philadelphia, a grown woman quite able to take care of myself. I didn't have to worry about anyone putting me out in the street. Still, I had never forgiven Daddy for the way he treated me that night, and as Mommy and I stood in her living room, I realized that I'd never forgiven her, either, for not standing up for me more vigorously with Daddy. No. I wouldn't be staying at the house.

"Mommy," I said gently, "I have so much to do to get things together for Robby and me. I'd be on the phone and in and out of the house all the time. You'd never see me, anyway. Besides, Robby will be here. He's who you've missed anyway, right?" I said, attempting a joke I knew Mommy wouldn't find funny. However, my mother laughed a little and gave me a quick squeeze.

"Will you be here on Sunday for dinner? You haven't seen your father since you've been back."

I put my arms around my mother's waist and squeezed her right back. Although I wasn't sure if I was coming to dinner or not, I nodded my head yes and hurried toward the door. I didn't want things to get too sappy between us. In a weak moment, I might be tempted to lay my head on her shoulder and tell her about the illness I was hiding.

I looked for an apartment in a safe neighborhood, convenient to my office in center city, and found a place in the Queens Village neighborhood of South Philly. Queens Village, bounded on the east by the Philadelphia Waterfront, had grown over the centuries from being one of Philly's earliest settlements to one of the city's most upscale areas. The neighborhood certainly had its share of crime, given its proximity to South Street (the hippest street in town), which brought rowdy crowds into the neighborhood on the weekends, and to the Southwark public housing projects before they were torn down in 2000. But I felt certain that Queens Village was safer for Robby and me than some of the more drug and crime-ridden areas of the city.

Our new place was a modern two-bedroom apartment on the first floor of a converted three-story house at Third and Fitzwater only a few blocks from South Street. Robby and I had lived on South Street in the 1970s with my ex-husband Alexs, before moving to the Twin Cities. South Street had changed a lot since those days. While still a center for nightlife, much of the edgy feel the street was known for back then was gone. The Painted Bride Art Center, an alternative art space that occupied an old bridal salon in the 300 block of South, had moved north to Old City. Grendel's Lair, the raucous music and dance club at 500 South St, known for presenting some of the most eclectic music in the city, was closing, to be replaced by a Gap store.

While I was dismayed to see these changes to iconic South Street, after living in the primarily vanilla and staid Twin Cities for five years, I loved my new surroundings. Queens Village itself was also predominately White, but eventually, everybody, regardless of race, came to South Street just a few blocks away. Besides, despite the changes, there were still a few oases of "funk" and counterculture to be found in the area. The Garden of Letters bookstore stood defiantly at 527 South with the big iron lion still guarding the entrance and Nag Champa incense wafting out the door. One block down, the magical Eyes Gallery, which had been selling Latin America folk art, clothing, and jewelry since the 1960s, was still doing a brisk business, as was the legendary Jim's Steaks, famous for slathering their steak sandwiches with Cheese Whiz.

My job was only two miles from my new apartment, which meant I could walk to my office or take my choice of the buses running west on Lombard, Spruce, or Walnut Streets. I usually avoided the buses, using the walk as part of my fitness routine. A healthy heart would benefit any condition, right?

However, Robby wasn't at all happy about leaving his friends in Minneapolis/St. Paul. By fall, he was in a new high school and had made the soccer team. That accomplishment was tempered by the fact that the school was at least an hour's ride away on public transportation. Each day, Robby seemed less impressed with me and the choices I made for our lives. Our relationship had started to change in the Twin Cities once he hit his teens, but this move back to Philadelphia put even more distance and silence between us. Almost any conversation between us became an argument. I knew this kind of rift happened between parents and adolescents, but Robby's attitude toward me cut deep. We'd been close since the day he was born. I worried all the time about how he'd feel toward me if he knew I was keeping my illness from him.

One day, in a rare moment of candor, shortly after we'd settled in our new apartment, Robby said to me:

"You know I didn't want to leave Minnesota, but I thought that at least in Philly, I'd be able to spend more time with my dad."

His statement hung in the air as we both silently acknowledged his disappointment. I knew better than to say a word since I was not at all objective about Robby's relationship with his father. I could see my child was in pain but there was nothing I could do to make things better. He and his father would have to work out their relationship without me. Shortly after this conversation, my son announced he didn't want to be called Robby anymore.

"I'm Rob," he said.

I stared at my son more closely than I had in a while. He was growing up more quickly than I'd realized. I could see why he might not want to be called by his childhood nickname "Robby" anymore. I chose my words carefully when I answered him.

"Okay, Rob," I said. "I won't call you Robby anymore. But I might not always remember to call you Rob and reserve the right to call you by your whole name, 'Robert.' Okay?"

Rob stared back at me, seeming unsure about whether he wanted to agree to my compromise. After a few seconds, he nodded his head yes.

∼

MY SON, ROB, was smart, charming, and sophisticated for a kid his age. He was also beautiful, with a deep chocolate brown complexion and a head full of woolly hair. People were drawn to Rob, and he made new friends quickly in Philadelphia, many of whom I didn't know. More worrying to me, Rob began to spend more time out of the house than in. I silently hoped that I hadn't made a mistake bringing him back to Philadelphia where the streets were much more dangerous than they were in the Twin Cities. I was shocked one day when he said, "Mom, I have a job after school."

I almost fell on the floor. I disapproved vehemently. Insulted and angry, I let him know.

"Why in the world do you need a job?" I asked incredulously. "I work hard every day so you don't have to. Why do you need money? You're only fifteen. You should be studying after school, not working."

I could hear my voice rising to the point of hysteria. My dad used to tell us how hard he worked as a child, after school and on the weekends, to help support his brothers and sisters. *Don't you understand, I wanted to scream at him. There is no need for you to repeat this history!* I knew Rob wasn't thinking about history. He'd found another way to declare his independence from me.

In desperation, I thought about asking Daddy to talk some sense into his grandson. Daddy and Rob had a stronger relationship than I'd ever had with my father. I quickly decided against that strategy since honestly I wasn't sure what Daddy would tell him. My father believed in hard work more than he believed in a lot of things. He might think a job after school was good for Rob. I'd heard him say, "A little work ain't never hurt nobody." The last thing I needed was Daddy siding with my son against me.

There wasn't a thing I could do to stop Rob from working. I was at work myself when he got out of school and had little control over what he did with his time. Rob started working as an all-around helper at Chefs Gourmet Market on South Street. I'd go into the store from time to time to check on him. Sometimes he didn't know I was there. He seemed happy, but I hated to see him with a broom in his hands.

Eventually, I grudgingly accepted Rob's job. "There are worse things he could be doing after school," I told myself with resignation. Still, I worried about him constantly. I worried about his schoolwork, and I worried about him roaming around the city. Most days I crossed my heart, fingers, and toes and hoped for the best. I had no choice. I had to work.

After a year or so back in Philly, I finally did what I knew I needed to do. I found a doctor—Dr. Frankel, a well-regarded internist recommended by friends, to take care of me and Rob generally, but also to monitor my kidney disease. By the time I started seeing him, my blood pressure and cholesterol had become slightly elevated. He began treating me with medication for both, trying to keep the FSGS at bay.

"You look pretty healthy to me," Dr. Frankel would say with a chuckle when I saw him twice a year. I always found this comment a bit cavalier and annoying. I knew looks meant nothing. I'd looked healthy my entire life, but I still had FSGS. I couldn't relax until I received a call from his nurse a few days later with my lab results.

"Ms. Watson, everything looks good," she'd say in a singsong voice, pronouncing the word "good" like it has two syllables. "Your kidney function is normal, the same as last time. So, we'll see you in six months, okaaay?"

Sometimes, I allowed myself to feel hopeful. Between doctor's visits, I tried not to think about kidney disease. I tucked the letters FSGS away in the back of my brain where I could ignore them for a while. And why not? A famous nephrologist at the Mayo Clinic told me the FSGS might never progress enough to cause real damage to my kidneys. When I needed the reassurance, I repeated the words from Dr. Donadio's letter, "Your prognosis is very good." Maybe Donadio was right.

Fortunately, I loved my new job and was good at it. One of my responsibilities was to evaluate a college preparation project for Black and Latino students run by the City University of New York. My boss trusted me with the entire effort from data collection to writing the final report. I began to trust my skills. I was a good writer and diligent worker. With Rob spending so much time out of the house, I started going into the office on Saturdays and sometimes even Sundays. This only made things worse between Rob and me. The less time we spent together, the more tense things were.

One especially tense and hot summer day, I lost my temper when Rob wouldn't tell me where he'd been until the wee hours. I became so frustrated that I almost struck him. Fortunately, I had the good sense to lower my hand as quickly as I raised it. I remembered how my father's beatings had caused lasting resentment in me. "What is the matter with me?" I thought. "Am I working too hard? Am I still so stressed out from the move or the break-up of my marriage that I'm taking it out on my kid?" I knew those could very well be partial reasons for my short fuse. However, deep down inside I was also aware that the secret I carried was the real culprit. I never knew when or if the FSGS would strike, destroying my kidneys and possibly my life. I was never truly at peace.

Still, my career blossomed. In 1988, I was recruited by a Philadelphia-based, nationally regarded, social policy research firm that developed and analyzed programs for vulnerable youth. The work was personal to me. Where would I be without social policies designed to help young people who needed opportunities? My management skills, sharpened through years of simultaneously working, going to school, and raising a kid as a single parent, were a great benefit in my new job. However, my writing skill is what separated me from other talented staff. Promotions came quickly.

When Rob left for college in 1989, I moved to the Old City neighborhood in the northern-most part of Philadelphia's center city. The South Street area had lost its appeal to me. The almost nightly din was wearing my nerves to a frazzle. Rob introduced me to Old City after riding the # 57 bus through the area on his way to school. Despite our issues, Rob knew me better than anyone.

"You'll like this neighborhood," he said. "It's you."

He was right. I loved Old City's history and character. When I moved there, the streets were still dotted with old warehouses, factories, and artisan shops. These structures had hummed with activity during the 19th century, Philadelphia's manufacturing heyday. By the 1960s, as the city's industrial base declined, most of the manufacturing concerns ceased operations, leaving abandoned structures behind. Artists, many fleeing the increasing commercialization of South Street, recycled the buildings into living and performance spaces. By the '70s, developers were converting these historical structures into apartments, lofts, and condos. However, when I moved into my apartment at Bridgeview, the site of a former boilermaker at 315 New Street, the neighborhood was still a decade away from being over-run with commercial establishments, Gen-Xers, and weekend tourists.

I lived at Bridgeview for fifteen years: first in a tiny one-bedroom on the first floor and then in a slightly roomier two-bedroom on the third floor. In 1994, I bought a beauty with exposed brick, huge windows, and a view of the big, blue Benjamin Franklin Bridge for which the building was named. I loved the place. At Bridgeview, I came as close as I ever had to living the life I wanted.

In addition to working, I hung out with old friends and made new ones. I filled my home with art; expanded my jazz collection; enjoyed my work; and threw fabulous parties on the building's roof-top every July to celebrate my birthday. I enjoyed the company of lovers and learned to love my own company. I became a patron of the arts, began to write poetry, and had my first poetry reading at the Painted Bride Art Center which was right across the street from my condo. Three to four times a week, I worked out at the downtown YMCA on 15th and Arch streets before or after work. Yoga became a true passion and walking was my primary mode of getting around the city. I experimented with different forms of meditation to reduce stress and changed my diet to eliminate red meat, include more fruits and vegetables, and increase the amount of water I drank.

In the summer of 1992, during a routine office visit, Dr. Frankel suggested that I begin seeing a nephrologist. He explained that I was generally in good health except for an elevated cholesterol reading of 284 and that my kidney function remained normal with a creatinine of .9 milligrams. However, my lab reports since he'd begun treating me five years before, showed about the same percentage of protein in my urine.

"I'm pleased that the protein hasn't increased, Ms. Watson, but the measurements haven't decreased, either. I'm not a kidney specialist and I want you to have a nephrologist on hand who knows your case if you need one."

Listening to Dr. Frankel's words, tears sprung up behind my eyelids like they'd been in my eyes all the time, waiting for the opportunity to fall. I didn't even look up at the doctor, since I didn't want him to see me cry. I was a grown woman, after all, forty-one years old to be exact. I stared at the floor as I questioned him.

"Why are you telling me this now? What's changed? You say I'm doing fine. Why do I need another doctor in my life? Can't you continue to monitor me?"

My voice was rising and I could feel myself getting angry. Eventually, I looked up at Dr. Frankel and couldn't keep tears from falling onto my face. Frankel seemed astonished that I was so upset.

"Please, Ms. Watson," he said, sounding as alarmed as I was. "Don't get upset. You're doing remarkably well. You've been dealing with this disease for almost a decade and your condition is still stable. But I want you to get the best care possible and I've done all I can do. FSGS is a tricky disease. I've told you all along that your kidney function could begin to deteriorate at any point."

I wiped tears from my face and continued to stare at the doctor, but I wasn't listening to him closely. I was working hard to keep hold of my emotions so that I didn't have a full meltdown in his office. The doctor handed me a tissue and, at the same time, a page from his prescription pad where he'd scribbled out a name and number.

"I want you to see Michael Rudnick over at Graduate Hospital—18th and Lombard. He's one of the most brilliant nephrologists in the business. I'll still be involved in your care, Ms. Watson, but let's see what Dr. Rudnick has to say."

The problem was that I didn't want to hear what Dr. Rudnick had to say. As ridiculous as it sounds, I believed then that just seeing a nephrologist would cause my kidney function to deteriorate. I was sure I'd be tangled up in the medical system and never get out. Kidney failure would become a self-fulfilling prophecy.

I didn't take Dr. Frankel's advice immediately. I was too stubborn for that. Or maybe I was too scared, or too angry, or too ashamed of having this damn disease. Sometimes I felt all four emotions at once. I finally made an appointment to see Rudnick several months later in November, after a cold that lasted too long prompted me to action.

Dr. Rudnick was tall, thin, and somewhat brusque, and showed little desire for small talk. He was thorough, however, and in addition to taking blood and urine samples, poked, prodded, and questioned me about my medical history for an hour. His ears perked up when I mentioned intermittent joint pain in my left knee and hip.

"Have you ever been diagnosed with lupus?" he asked, squinting down at me. "I'm curious if you may have a form of systemic lupus erythematosus, which can attack the kidneys."

I stared back at him blankly and shook my head no. For heaven's sake, I certainly didn't want any more ailments.

"Hmm," Rudnick grunted, standing over me with his arms folded across his wiry frame. He seemed genuinely excited about another line of inquiry that might explain why a healthy young woman like me might develop FSGS.

"Well," he said after a moment in thought. "We can follow that possibility in future evaluations."

However, like other doctors I'd seen, Rudnick concluded that he wouldn't recommend any specific treatment at that time.

"I've seen your records, Ms. Watson, and based on my current evaluation, your kidney function is well preserved—your creatinine is 1.1 milligrams and the amount of protein present in your urine is unchanged. Of course, I want to continue to follow you and would like to see you again in about six months.

If your renal function has worsened, I'll consider another renal biopsy to compare with the tissue from the 1984 sample."

Blah, blah blah I thought to myself as I pretended to listen to Dr. Rudnick. For the past eight years, I'd heard the same words from doctors. Rudnick was the third doctor to tell me: You have protein in your urine, but your kidney function is good. Fine. If my kidney function was good, that was all I cared about. I tuned back into Rudnick's drone in time to hear him say something about me seeing a rheumatologist about the possibility of lupus in my case, but my mind was already out the door. I had no intention of seeing another specialist unless I truly needed one. The last thing I wanted was to become a professional patient.

Walking out of Dr. Rudnick's office that afternoon in November 1992 I decided, *life is short.* If my kidney function is good, why should I need so much doctoring? I'm going to be as happy as I can be under the circumstances. I'll take as good care of myself for as long as I can, without becoming part of the medical machine.

The faster I walked and the further I got from the doctor's office, the more determined I became. By the time I'd walked the two miles back to my Old City apartment, I'd decided not to make a follow-up appointment with Rudnick. I didn't need him "following" me. I didn't know if that decision was smart or not. I only knew what felt right to me at that moment.

Dr. Frankel, my internist, scoffed at my decision not to see the nephrologist regularly but agreed to evaluate my kidney function on an annual basis. For my part, I focused on healthy living more than ever—determined to halt, if not reverse the effects of FSGS on my body. I took my blood pressure and cholesterol medicines religiously. I meditated regularly and even found a natural health care practitioner who sold me herbal teas that were supposed to help normalize my kidney function.

I also began to see a chiropractor weekly. My first visit to was for chronic neck pain, most likely a result of hunching over a computer for years. However, he convinced me that the chiropractic treatment helped the entire body and could help my kidneys. Neither the chiropractor nor natural health practitioner was covered by my insurance, but I happily paid for these services out of pocket. I would have paid any amount to have my good health back.

During the early to late 1990s, as I did what I could to take care of my health, I also took great pleasure in pampering myself. As far as I was concerned, I deserved the good life. Who knew what was coming? After paying my bills and saving for what I thought could be a bumpy future, I spent liberally on clothes, haircuts, nails, facials, and other self-care. I was determined to look and feel as well as I could. Taking care of myself was something I could control, and I needed to be in control of something. Everything looked good, until it didn't.

One day, in the spring of 1998, I found myself sitting at my kitchen counter with a cup of oolong tea in my hand and a knot in my stomach. I'd seen Frankel for a check-up a few days before. Now I was nervous because the nurse usually called within a day or two of the visits. I never expected bad news, nevertheless, I found it hard to stay calm.

"Girl, you've lived with this disease for fourteen years and nothing's happened," I'd whisper to myself. "You're fine. Breathe in, breathe out."

I'd been taking yoga classes for years now and had learned

to use deep breathing as a relaxation technique. Sometimes this worked.

The telephone rang and I took one last deep breath in through my nose and let it out slowly through my mouth.

"Hello, Dine Watson," I said, trying to sound like I was answering a routine business call.

"Hello, is this Ms. Watson?"

My breath caught in my throat. This wasn't the nurse's singsongy voice at all. The doctor himself was calling. Something was wrong.

"Yes," I said, holding on tightly to the counter's ledge. "This is Ms. Watson."

"Hello, Ms. Watson, this is Dr. Frankel." This time there was no chuckling and no banter about my looks. The good doctor was playing things entirely straight. I picked up my cup and took a sip. The tea was cold, always a bad sign in my book.

"Ms. Watson, I think it's time for you to see Dr. Rudnick again. Your creatinine level is creeping up."

I didn't hear another word he said.

Chapter Two:
YOUR CREATININE LEVEL IS CREEPING UP

I had the blues and couldn't shake them.

Every day since Dr. Frank's call had been a "blue day." I couldn't get his fateful words out of my head.

Fortunately, I wasn't stupid. Say what you want about the Hayes clan. We aren't stupid people—stubborn, prideful, and even reckless sometimes. But my good sense, my survival instinct told me that I shouldn't ignore Dr. Frankel's recommendation this time. Wearily, a few weeks after Frankel's call, I pulled myself together and made an appointment to see Dr. Rudnick, the brilliant nephrologist.

The morning I arrived at Dr. Rudnick's office, I was the only patient sitting in the waiting room. The place was eerily quiet. Rudnick startled me when he seemed to appear out of nowhere.

"Well, Ms. Watson, as I live and breathe," he said with what looked like a slight smirk across his thin face. Despite his remark, Rudnick didn't seem surprised to see me. He sounded sarcastic and I got the feeling that he'd always expected me to walk back into his office one day. Score one for the doctor. I stuttered, for a few seconds trying to get my words together, then gave up on speaking and nodded politely. The man intimidated me. Just being in his office made me sweat. My underwear began to stick to my crotch. My feet felt glued to the floor. I managed to pull myself up, however, when Rudnick waved at me. "Why don't you go on into the examining room and get undressed from the waist up."

Sure thing, I thought. I wanted nothing more than to get this whole episode over with.

"It's been a while since I've seen you, Ms. Watson," Rudnick said, towering over me. "You're an interesting case. I thought I would have the opportunity to follow your condition. How are you doing?"

I'm an interesting case, I thought. What the hell does that mean? I wasn't sure I wanted to know. As for his question, "how are you doing?" I could hardly keep up with my feelings these days. I'd felt fine until a few months ago when Frankel told me that my creatinine was rising. Since then, I'd been a nervous wreck. Today was no different. All I could do was give Rudnick a pat answer.

"I'm doing okay, Doctor," I said quietly, unable to add any enthusiasm to my voice.

"Why haven't I seen you in such a long time? Why haven't you come in?" Rudnick pressed, staring at me with his arms folded across his chest.

Again, I felt intimidated. Here I was sitting in the examining room, half-dressed, with him staring down at me. I searched for a suitable answer to his question. In my nervousness, the absolute truth came tumbling out of my mouth. "Honestly, Dr. Rudnick, I was tired of coming to the doctor. You are the fourth doctor I've seen for FSGS and every single one, including you, has told me the same thing… you're doing well; your condition is stable… so I didn't see the need to keep coming to doctors. I just want to live my life."

Rudnick stared at me intensely for a moment and looked as if he was about to give me a lecture, then he turned abruptly as if he decided not to try and reason with me. He reached for a standing blood pressure monitor in the corner of the exam room.

"Hand me your arm please and just breathe normally," Rudnick said in a monotone, as I stared up into the ceiling, only turning to look at him when I heard the cup deflate. I couldn't see the reading on the monitor, but the frown forming at the corner of Rudnick's mouth told me the number wasn't good.

"170/90, that's pretty high, Ms. Watson," he said. "I don't recall your pressures being that high. Did you take your medication today?"

"I take my medicine religiously," I answered. The high blood pressure reading didn't make me happy either. For as long as doctors had been taking my pressure, a high reading could ruin my day.

"Do you take your pressures at home?" Rudnick asked. "What are they like at home?"

His question made me feel defensive as if I were being chastised.

"No, I don't take them home," I said, my voice rising a little. "I see Dr. Frankel twice a year and rely on his readings. They've always been pretty good. Why would my pressure be that high?" I asked with annoyance. "I take my medicine and work out 3-4 times a week. I'm not overweight and I eat healthily. Can you take my pressure again please?"

Without hesitation, Rudnick nodded his head. "Why don't you stand up. We'll see what your standing pressure is like."

I stood up obediently, clutching the paper gown to me with my left arm as I again held out my right. My heart pounded as I watched Rudnick's face and felt the cup's tight squeeze. I could see that he still wasn't pleased.

"No change, Ms. Watson. Your pressure is still 170/90. Let me look at your eyes," he said, picking up a scope of some kind from a side table. "Your pressure is high, and I want to make sure your retinas look okay. Just relax."

"Relax, relax," I whispered to myself, but the longer I stood there in that skimpy gown the more anxious I felt. Besides, I was getting cold and beginning to shiver.

Dr. Rudnick lowered the scope and looked at me somewhat sympathetically. "Your eyes look fine Ms. Watson. Why don't you get dressed and sit here quietly for a few moments? We can postpone the rest of your exam till next time, but I'll come back and check your pressure one more time."

Rudnick surprised me by patting my arm as he walked out of the room. Honestly, I was glad to have a personal gesture from him. If I was going to have to see him regularly, I wanted to know that I wasn't just an "interesting case" to him.

Wearily, I pulled my shirt over my head, lay down on the examining table, and closed my eyes. The sky-high blood pressure numbers scared me. A rare, hopeful thought, however, crossed my mind. Maybe I was suffering from the white coat effect. Once, after an uncharacteristically high blood pressure reading in his office, Dr. Frankel explained that sometimes patients' subconscious fear of doctors (white coats) is reflected in higher-than-normal blood pressure readings. Dr. Rudnick did scare me after all. But 170/90 was very high for me. Maybe after all these years, my kidneys were finally giving out. Maybe FSGS was my fate and there was nothing I could do about it.

My blues were turning bluer and sinking deeper when Rudnick came back into the room and slowly put the cuff back on my arm.

"Breathe normally," he said. "Just relax your arm." I tried to do both.

This time the reading was lower. "140/85," he said. "You've been still for a while, so your pressure's gone down some, but it's still higher than I'd like. Look, Ms. Watson, you're in remarkably good shape, but you have kidney disease. According to the labs I got from Dr. Frankel, your creatinine level is rising, and your blood pressure is likely to rise too. That's what happens." He gave me one of those matter-of-fact looks that I hated.

I left Rudnick's office that day with a prescription for Vasotec, a blood pressure medication that he described as a miracle drug.

"I'm hoping that the Vasotec will help bring your pressure down and reduce the amount of protein in your urine." He also handed me a portable blood pressure machine about the size of an old fashion cassette player.

"I want you to keep this machine on for 24 hours and return it to me within a few days," Dr. Rudnick ordered. "I'd like to see your readings at different times of the day and night. This will tell me what your blood pressure is really doing."

Before I could walk out of the door, he handed me a lab slip. How could I forget that I couldn't leave the hospital without peeing in a cup or having a needle jammed into my arm for blood work?

Walking out of the office, my heart felt heavier than the clunky machine I carried. I felt like a chump. For as long as I could remember, I'd tried to take care of my body. Now, one of my biggest fears was becoming a reality. I was being sucked into the medical system.

I returned the blood pressure machine to Rudnick's office in a few days, and two weeks later, was back in his tiny examining room. Unfortunately, according to readings from the machine, my blood pressure was high even when I was sleeping. I felt disgusted and angry with my body. If my blood pressure wouldn't behave when I was asleep, what could I do about it?

"I'm taking the Vasotec as you prescribed," I responded, shrugging my shoulders.

"I'm sure, I'm sure, Ms. Watson," he responded quickly. "Let's see what your pressure is now that you've been taking this new medication for a few weeks." When Rudnick nodded affirmatively as the cuff deflated, I let out a sigh of relief.

"Very good, Ms. Watson," he said, almost smiling. "130/80. The Vasotec is working. I told you it's a miracle drug. Now leave a urine sample for me at the lab and we'll see if the proteinuria has decreased. A call from the good doctor a few days later had me dancing in my kitchen.

"Ms. Watson, you've had an excellent response from the Vasotec, not just in terms of reducing your hypertension, but in decreasing the proteinuria. Why don't you continue the Vasotec and come back in four months for a blood pressure check and labs. Okay, Ms. Watson? Have a good summer."

I don't know if I said goodbye to Dr. Rudnick or thanked him for this good news. I only remember dropping the phone onto my kitchen counter and hopping across the floor to a cha-cha beat. A feeling of pure joy rushed through my whole body. Could it be that I was going to be okay? Maybe, just maybe, all the care I'd taken—exercise, yoga, meditation, dietary changes—and, yes, miracle drugs, were finally working. The relief was unexplainable. At forty-six-years old someone had commuted my death sentence. I exhaled.

When I returned to Dr. Rudnick's office for my September appointment, I was in decent spirits. Rudnick had wished me a good summer and I'd had one, celebrating my 47th birthday with a big "soiree" on the rooftop of my condo building. All I wanted now was a good report from my nephrologist.

As usual, butterflies fluttered around in my stomach as I approached the doctor's office, but I was in no way prepared for the disappointment waiting for me. Despite the miracle drug, my sitting blood pressure had soared back up to dangerously elevated levels and my standing pressure was only moderately better. Rudnick didn't have to tell me that the reading wasn't a good sign. In fact, he and I didn't bother to talk much at all during that visit as if we were both depressed that our efforts weren't yielding the expected results. What the hell, I wondered. How could I feel so good when such bad things were going on inside my body? Should I have known better than to think I might be okay? Who's to say? As another doctor once told me, "Sometimes your body lets you down." Without looking at me directly Rudnick began scribbling on his prescription pad.

"I'm going to increase the Vasotec to see if we can stabilize your pressure. Today's labs will tell us what's going on with your creatinine. I'm also going to go ahead and increase the Lipitor for your cholesterol."

Rudnick finally looked at me as he handed me the prescriptions and lab slips. His eyes looked weary—like he'd given out a lot of bad news that day. For the first time, I got a sense of how much Rudnick genuinely cared about his patients. Maybe the gruff exterior he presented on most days was his way of protecting himself from what could be a brutal job. I felt for the man.

"I'll call in a few days with your lab results," he said, sounding exhausted. "They'll tell us if we need to schedule another biopsy. I don't want to do the biopsy unless it's necessary. Biopsies have their risks too."

The labs showed that there was blood in my urine. As a female, I'd seen plenty of blood in the toilet over the years, but the thought of actually peeing blood made me shiver.

"That can't be a good sign," I whispered under my breath as Rudnick continued with the unwelcome news.

"You're also spilling more protein into your urine and your creatinine level is up significantly."

I knew that my creatinine level revealed how well my kidneys were working.

"What is my creatinine level now, Doctor?" I asked, the nervousness in my stomach, finding its way into my voice.

"Your creatinine is 3.0 mgs, Ms. Watson, up from 1.2 just a few months ago."

I fell silent. In fact, for a moment I don't think I could say, hear or feel anything. Later, I remember thinking that Rudnick's comment about my rising creatinine had sent me into a state of suspended animation, where nothing—not pain, disappointment, or fear, could reach me. Then I heard Rudnick's voice, filling the silence, bringing me back to our conversation.

"Ms. Watson, I think it's time for another biopsy. We need to see if there's more scarring of your kidneys. Given the increased protein and the rise in your creatinine level, I suspect we'll see more scarring."

When I still didn't respond, Rudnick kept talking. "Don't worry, Ms. Watson. You've been through this before. A biopsy is very minor surgery. My colleague, Rafe Cohen, can handle the procedure right here in our office. I'll have someone call you about dates. Okay, Ms. Watson?"

I could hear every word Dr. Rudnick was saying and could tell that he was waiting for me to respond. Again, my mind went elsewhere. This time, I'd traveled back to 1984—fourteen years ago— to Minneapolis and my first biopsy. My friend Jeanie had been with me and held my hand through the ordeal. This time I'd be alone. I didn't want or need anyone with me.

∼

ON THE SATURDAY after my dispiriting appointment with Dr. Rudnick, the sky was gloomy and portending rain. Still, I walked the mile from my apartment in Old City to the Reading Terminal at 11th and Arch. The Terminal is one of my favorite places in the city. Maybe the walk, part of my exercise regimen, and the colorful, crowded hustle of the market would cheer me up. At the market, I bought lavender alstroemeria for my dining room table and chicken lo mein from the San Kee Peking Duck stall. I knew about the lo mein's salt content and the possible repercussions for my kidney condition, but I had been limiting my salt content all week, and dammit, I could smell those noodles. I was going to have lo mein today and worry about the sodium tomorrow.

Walking back home to my apartment under the increasingly threatening sky, I felt lonely and more than a little tired. The tiredness annoyed me more than the loneliness since I suspected the FSGS of sapping my energy. FSGS. Fuck Shit Goddam this Shit.

It couldn't be more than one o'clock in the afternoon and I shouldn't feel so drained. And since when didn't I enjoy my own company? Fueled only by the thought of diving into my delicious lunch, I soldiered on.

The lo mein was scrumptious, especially after I added a few dashes of garlic, onion, smoked paprika, and truth be told, more soy sauce. I always seasoned take-out food to suit my tastes, but more sauce? More sodium? What was wrong with me? Frankly,

I knew what was wrong with me and eating the salty lo mein would probably only make things worse. I'd sunk back into the deep, blue funk I'd woken up with and my usually enjoyable trip to the Reading Terminal hadn't helped at all. When I felt this bad, my carefully honed good eating habits deserted me.

    I sat at my kitchen counter and stared at the view outside the big picture window in my living room. I let myself get lost in the cars speeding across the Ben Franklin bridge from Philly to New Jersey. Where are all these people going? I wondered. The Camden Aquarium? Cherry Hill Mall? Corrine's Soul Food place on Haddon Avenue? I wondered how many of them had heard of FSGS. For the first time that day, I laughed. What a crazy thought. Maybe this FSGS was affecting my brain. Maybe I was losing my mind as well as my body.

    When I finally turned around to check the time, the clock on the microwave read 4:30. My day was almost over. Remnants from the lunch I'd slurped down—the empty aluminum foil container, a crumpled napkin, and a plastic carry bag—were still sitting on the kitchen counter. The place smelled like soy sauce, but I couldn't make myself get up from the stool and clean up. So what? Who cares if my kitchen is a mess? Apparently, my body was a mess too. In fact, the whole world seemed a mess. All I had to do was look at the news. So far in 1998, students in Jonesboro, Arkansas, and Springfield, Oregon had taken guns to school and killed fellow students. In June, a White supremacist had dragged James Byrd for three miles behind a pickup truck simply because he was Black. In August of this year, 200 people were killed when two US embassies were bombed in Dar Es Salaam, Tanzania, and Nairobi, Kenya. My messy kitchen wasn't hurting anybody.

    The phone was ringing. I looked over at the caller ID.

Mommy was calling. Ugh. I loved my mother but didn't want to talk. I stared at the phone for a while, but on the fourth ring reluctantly decided to pick it up. I'd feel guilty for the rest of the day if I didn't answer.

"Hi Mommy," I said, thankful that she couldn't see my kitchen.

"Hi, B," she said. Her voice sounded small and weary. Before I could ask what was wrong and prepare myself for her answer, Mommy launched right in.

"Your father passed out yesterday and is in the hospital. The doctor says he has a carotid artery, a complication from his diabetes. Daddy wants everybody up at the hospital tomorrow."

"What?" I almost shouted in disbelief. "Daddy's in the hospital? Good Grief! Mommy, when did all this happen? How's Daddy doing?"

Mommy sounded exasperated. "Like I told you B, he passed out yesterday. He's in the hospital and wants all the children up there tomorrow. Alice and your brother Jerry are coming down from New York."

My heart flip flopped. Why does he want all of us there? What's going on?

"Mommy, how sick is Daddy? How serious is this?"

My mother was silent for a moment as if she needed time to think about how to answer me.

"B, he's pretty sick," she said, sounding sick herself. "At some point, he needs surgery to unblock the carotid artery—this is all related to your father's diabetes. He's tried to hide it, but can't you tell he hasn't been feeling well?"

My mother's question stopped me cold. When was the last time I'd seen Daddy? When was the last time I actually looked at him? I couldn't remember.

"He wants us there tomorrow?" I asked, searching my mental calendar for the other things I was sure I had to do on Sunday.

"Yes, tomorrow," Mommy said. "You'll be there, right?"

Mommy was right to try to pin me down. The truth was, I didn't see my parents much. We lived at opposite ends of the city—Mommy and Daddy lived uptown, close to the northern end of Philadelphia; while I lived downtown, close to the Delaware River on the southern end. I usually went uptown to see them when the extended family gathered at their house for special occasions, but they rarely came downtown to see me. Occasionally, Daddy would drop by my place unannounced, but my reception was often chilly and unwelcoming. Why couldn't he call and let me know he was coming or better yet, ask if I was up for a visit? The truth is, I'd never forgiven Daddy for so much—his controlling personality and harshness, his reaction to my teenage pregnancy.

I could recall every slap and slight from him with no trouble. All that ugliness hung in the air between us whenever we saw each other. I did what I could to keep our visits to a minimum. When I didn't answer my mother's question, she kept on talking. "I think he's going to be all right, though. I've been on my knees praying every day. The doctor who'll do Dad's surgery is Black and that gives your father a lot of confidence."

"Really, Mommy?" I said in a snide tone I rarely used in speaking to either of my parents. "Are you telling me that Daddy has confidence in this doctor because the man is Black? Are you kidding me?"

My mother sounded defensive when she responded. "Well, not only because he's Black, but you know your father."

Yes, I knew my father. Daddy was a race man. He loved

Black achievers and was probably mightily impressed by that Black doctor in his white coat.

All the talk about doctors and surgery was making me nervous. I, too, might be having surgery soon—a kidney transplant—something Mommy or anyone else in the family didn't know anything about yet.

"Please, Mommy," I said, more impatiently than I meant to sound. "Just tell me what hospital Daddy is in and I'll be there." I was immediately sorry for my tone of voice. None of this was Mommy's fault.

"He's up at Einstein, sweetheart. Brother Jerry said he'll be down around two o'clock."

I took a deep breath. "Okay," I said as calmly as I could manage. "I'll meet everyone at Einstein around 2:00. See you tomorrow."

I arrived at Einstein Hospital at around two o'clock p.m. on Sunday, just as Mommy had asked. Daddy was sitting up in a hospital bed surrounded by family: my four siblings—Baby Alice, Judy, Linda, and Brother Jerry, and several grandchildren. I exchanged glances with each of my siblings. I also saw a look of foreboding in their eyes. Every one of my siblings seemed to be thinking what I was thinking. Daddy was seriously ill. Why else would he have called us all here?

A white curtain separated Daddy from another patient who was moaning as if he was in a great deal of pain. On our side of the curtain, everyone including Daddy was laughing and joking as if they were at a party instead of in a hospital room. I waved at Rob, who was on the far side of the bed, and greeted my nieces and nephews with hugs and kisses before I took a good look at Daddy. I was surprised at how good he looked. I couldn't remember when I'd last seen him look so happy. He seemed ecstatic to have everyone gathered around him. Daddy was a lot of things, but I had to admit that first and foremost, he was a family man, even if I didn't always like the way he showed it. I took a deep breath and made my way to the head of the bed.

"Hi Pop," I said trying to sound casual.

"Hey B.B," he said, smiling and looking straight at me. I felt like he was trying to communicate a private message to me that I couldn't quite decipher. Bending over the bed, I gave Daddy a hug and a kiss on the cheek. He didn't resist. Daddy and I never hugged, much less kissed. I once asked him why he never hugged me and my siblings. He vaguely mentioned incest in his family when he was growing up, as the reason he never wanted to get too physically close to his daughters. I never pressed for details, but since he was lying in bed sick and couldn't stop me, I took the liberty of hugging him now. I was shocked by how frail he felt. His ribs were poking through his skin.

I stepped back from the bed to let one of the grandchildren move closer to Daddy. "I'll come back in a few days," I told myself. I'll come back when I can talk with Daddy alone and find out exactly what's going on. I looked around the room again to see if I could make eye contact with Robert or one of my siblings again to see if I could read their thoughts, but every eye was trained on Daddy. The laughing and talking continued. So did the moaning from behind the curtain.

No one seemed to want to leave Daddy's hospital room that Sunday afternoon, but around four o'clock my father started to doze. We all took turns saying our goodbyes with Daddy accepting hugs from everyone. When did all this start, I wondered. The Bernard Hayes I grew up with was not a hugger. I chose not to hug Daddy this time but kissed him on the forehead. I couldn't bear to feel his frail body again. He'd drifted off before I left his bedside.

Robert was waiting for me in the hospital hallway. With all the family crammed inside Daddy's room, we'd hardly had a chance to say hello. I quickly looked him up and down, so he wouldn't think I was giving him the motherly "once over." Frankly, I was admiring him. My son was a beautiful 50/50 combination of my father and his father. Sometimes I just needed to look at this child I had given birth to. I leaned into Rob as he put his arm around me.

"Are you coming back to the house, Ma?" he asked. "I hear Aunt Lin has ordered fish from that Muslim place we like. You look like you could use a meal."

Robert's comment about my looks startled me. How did I look? I constantly worried about looking ill, especially to my son, who had no idea what was going on with me. I didn't feel hungry, although I was tempted by the fish. I knew the Muslim takeout that Rob was talking about, and their fried fish was almost as good as Daddy's. But I demurred. The afternoon had taken a toll. Besides my biopsy was scheduled for Tuesday and I was worried. Weariness and worry, not hunger, was what my son saw in my face.

"No, son. I think I'm going to head back home. I have work to do," I lied. "Go on and catch up with your cousins. Make my excuses. Kiss Gram and eat some fish for me."

Robert stared at me for a moment as if deciding whether to press me, then said, "Okay, Ma, but at least let me walk you to the subway. Pop would kill me if I didn't at least do that."

Robert was right. My father had taught him the old-school value of looking out for the women in the family. We walked up to the Olney Avenue subway stop and passed the red brick wall of the Philadelphia High School for Girls, from where I'd graduated in 1969. "How many years ago was that?" I asked myself, trying to count the years in my head. No matter. The only thing that mattered right then was that I was walking down the street with my son—my son who'd been the focus of my life since I was a girl; my son, who had no idea how sick I was.

∞

As Rudnick suspected, the biopsy showed increased scarring in my kidneys. About two weeks after the procedure, I received a copy of the biopsy report from him, containing the pathologist's findings. The report was full of medical terminology that was difficult for me to understand, such as *globally sclerotic glomeruli, segmental scars and moderate to focally severe fibrosis, and tubular atrophy*. Still, I had enough sense to know that the report didn't contain good news. On my next visit, Rudnick, never one for subtleties, gave me the bottom line.

"Ms. Watson," he said dryly, staring at the report, "This biopsy indicates that the FSGS is advancing. The increased scarring correlates with the rising creatinine levels and increased proteinuria shown in your labs."

I heard Dr. Rudnick's voice, but for some reason I was fixated on the claustrophobic examining room we were in. Why are we always in this room, I thought. There was hardly enough space in there for the examining table and one hard plastic chair. Shouldn't a brilliant doctor have an office where he can talk to people after examining them? The news was bad enough without having to sit in that depressing little closet. However, there was no escaping Rudnick's words, which seemed to bounce off the walls in the increasingly airless room.

"We'll keep you on the Vasotec and the Lipitor, Ms. Watson," he continued. "FSGS is a terrible disease. If your creatinine level continues to rise, I suspect you'll need dialysis or a transplant in about a year. I'd advise you to start thinking about donors, but let's see what happens."

Chapter Three:
MAY DAY! MAY DAY!

Daddy died on Saturday, May 1, 1999. He'd entered the hospital for surgery to repair a blocked artery in his neck. I was prepared for him to be weak, frail, and even a little helpless after the surgery, but I was sure I'd have more time with him. I thought we'd have an honest talk and maybe reconcile things between us. I was even thinking of telling him my secret.

However, Daddy had a stroke after the surgery and went into a coma. He never woke up. I never got to talk to him as I'd planned to. When I went up to the hospital to visit him after the surgery, the nurses allowed me to see his big, bloated body through a glass window of the intensive care unit. The man I saw looked nothing like my father.

Daddy's dead? How can Daddy be dead? We weren't finished. Me and Daddy were supposed to have more time…a chance to talk. He was supposed to finally say he loved me, was proud of me, that he was sorry for…so many things. Daddy can't be gone. I never got a chance to tell him that I was sick. That I needed him here. That I needed his help.

We buried Daddy on the Friday after he died. Before I even arrived at the church for the funeral service, I was worn out with sorrow and stress. The last three weeks in a row had been woefully sad: first, the call from Mommy telling me that Daddy was in the hospital, then Daddy's death, now the funeral. I felt buffeted by ill winds. What the hell would come next? Dialysis? A transplant? My own death?

"Hush," I whispered aloud to myself. "Today is not about you, Dine. Daddy is the one who died."

I stared at my face one more time in the mirror before walking out of my front door. The bags under my eyes were more noticeable than usual. Too bad I never learned to use concealer. I hated those dark circles. They made me look tired, even ill. In fact, I thought to myself, today could be the day, that these dark circles betray me—give away my secret.

What's more, I was terrified. As I stared in the mirror, I found myself wishing for religion—a faith or belief system, anything to hold onto. Frankly, I'd never believed in much of anything I couldn't see with my own two eyes and had never been able to fake religious piety. I didn't absorb the dousing of Christianity my siblings and I were exposed to every Sunday at Tindley Temple Methodist Church.

Tindley, a great stone edifice on the corner of Broad and Fitzwater, around the corner from our house on Montrose Street, was one of the premier churches in Philadelphia for Blacks to worship on Sunday morning. The founder, Charles Albert Tindley, known in his day as "The Prince of Preachers," was a prolific composer of gospel hymns, many of which can still be found in church hymnals, regardless of denomination. In fact, back in the day, Tindley Temple was home to a large and proud congregation of the high and the low—judges, doctors, lawyers, teachers, and other professionals from Philadelphia's Black upper and middle classes, as well as struggling yet aspiring families like mine.

As far as my parents were concerned, anytime we weren't in school or doing homework was a good time to be in church. I believe keeping us "churched" was part of my parent's child-rearing strategy. They were hell-bent on making sure "y'all don't turn out like all these other kids up and down this block," as Daddy used to say—which meant assuring that none of their girls ended up pregnant and my brother didn't go to jail. Friday night was choir rehearsal; Saturday afternoon my sisters and I went to Brownie and Girls Scout meetings. Depending on the Sunday morning, we were either singing in the junior choir, ushering congregants to their pews, or sitting in the pews ourselves. Sunday afternoon meant Sunday School where we studied the Bible, and afterward, Methodist Youth Fellowship, where we learned about the responsibilities of being young Christians. In the summertime, when school was out, we attended Tindley Temple's Vacation Bible School. What's more, Mommy taught Sunday School every Sunday.

While Daddy insisted that his five children attend church every Sunday, he did not go to church himself. Sunday was Daddy's day to lie on the fold-out couch in the living room, also where he and Mommy slept every night, and watch sports after a week of back-breaking work on the construction site. But he didn't just lie around on Sundays. While the rest of the family was at church, Daddy moved between watching sports in the living room and cooking ham, chicken, or roast beef with all the trimmings for Sunday dinner. After dinner, he'd go right back to the couch to watch the evening news. Church did not fit into Daddy's day of rest.

While I went to church with the rest of the family and still know almost every song in the Methodist hymnal, traditional organized religion didn't take root in me as it did in my sisters, all three of whom are still observant Christians. Baby Alice is now a devout Seventh Day Adventist, Judith married a minister and sings God's praises in her church choir every Sunday, Linda and her husband are evangelicals, and my brother Jerry considers himself a Christian, even if he doesn't go to church every Sunday. While I remain the outlier among my siblings as far as traditional religion is concerned, on the morning of my father's funeral I wondered how it would feel if I could, like the old Methodist hymn said, "take my burden to the Lord and leave it there."

Daddy was "laid out" at Tindley Temple where he rarely set foot. I hadn't been back in the church in years, but the sanctuary still looked the same—the massive stained-glass windows, the long, sturdy, wooden pews, the royal looking red velvet coverings on the pulpit, the massive pipes of the magnificent Moller organ that sounded like a roll of heavenly thunder. I had forgotten the grandeur of my childhood church. *If I were ever going to be "saved," it would have happened in this place,* I thought.

About 200 mourners—family, friends, and acquaintances attended the service—a respectable number—but the vastness of the church sanctuary made the crowd seem smaller. The service itself was very dignified, with none of the loud wailing that I was used to hearing at other family funerals. The most notable noise came from Mommy sitting with my brother Jerry in the first pew, moaning and calling out my father's name repeatedly, "Bernard, Bernard, Bernard."

Don't get me wrong, people shed tears. Uncle Walter, who wasn't my father's blood brother, but his best friend from boyhood, was so choked up he could barely speak the "words of comfort" he'd been asked to make. Standing at the pulpit, he seemed unable to hold up his more than six-foot frame and looked exactly like who he was— a man who lost his best friend.

For a few seconds Uncle Walt stood at the pulpit in silence, at a loss for words. Finally, he said quietly, "Me and Bernard never had any trouble, we just never had any trouble." Then he shrugged his sloping shoulders and took his seat.

Uncle Walt's words stuck in my ears. "Me and Bernard never had any trouble." *How could that be*? I thought. No trouble? Never? I was Bernard's daughter, his namesake, the one everybody said was so much like him for God's sake, and he and I had plenty of trouble.

Sitting there in the church pew, I tried to pay attention to the ongoing service. A minister was in the pulpit speaking fervently, reading a Bible verse that I'm sure had some relationship to my father, and I should have been listening. But Uncle Walt had presented a picture of Daddy that I couldn't reconcile. No trouble. Wow! For as long as I could recall, Daddy had seemed like nothing but trouble for me. Yes, he'd fed, housed, clothed, and even named me, but he also yelled at me, cursed me, beat me, called me a whore, and caused me to leave home. Out of all his children, I always felt like I got the worst treatment from Daddy. Was it because I stood up to him, or jumped between him and Mommy when he raised his hand to slap her. Daddy? No trouble?

For the first time since my father's death, I felt tears on my face. I wasn't crying as much about his death as I was about the man I'd never known, the man my Uncle Walt was describing. Walter and Bernard had been boyhood friends. Maybe Uncle Walter had known a different Bernard.

Years after Daddy died, my sister Linda, found a yellow legal pad in his bedroom on which my father had told the story of his childhood. In his distinct, careful, handwriting Daddy began:

At this day and time in my life, I am sixty-three years old and have just retired from work, September 1990. Ladies and Gentlemen, I am writing this short history about myself while I am in sound mind and body. I hope these few words will give most of you some insight on what kind of person I am and was and some of the circumstances that made me this way.

Reading his story, I understood from his own words that my father never had much of a childhood. At ten years old he worked at a corner store and delivered newspapers after school and on Saturdays, to help support his family. When my father was twelve, his father left the family, leaving behind my Grandma Daisy and nine kids. Daddy had no choice but to become a major breadwinner. He wrote:

I was going to Jr. High school, delivering papers in the evenings, and working on Saturdays in a clothing factory. There my job was to clean the floors, oil the sewing machines, and help the layout men roll cloth and cut patterns for the pants, shirts, and dresses.

He also wrote of being the child his mother depended on most, of watching his mother change from being "a lady" to a "tough hardened woman," and of growing to despise his own father.

As I sat in the pew, head lowered, lost in my father's boyhood, I saw a vision of my father as a boy. The boy's face was determined, willful, almost defiant, a look I'd seen on my son Robert's face when he was angry, or on my brother Jerry's face when he was talking about something difficult. I'd even seen the same look on my own face once too often. I couldn't stop my tears.

As I wiped my face, I looked up just in time to see Uncle George, my father's only living brother, walking to the front of the church. While planning the funeral, my siblings and I wondered if we would see Uncle George, since he and Daddy feuded constantly and were estranged when Daddy died. The Hayes clan was known for its strong family resemblance, but Daddy and his brother George, the sibling he was closest to in age, looked like twins. When my Uncle George returned to his seat after viewing his brother's body, a thunderstorm raged across his face. Watching him cry so openly was like seeing my father with a face full of tears—something I'd never seen and could hardly bear to watch that day. I caught my uncle's eye as he passed my pew, and he managed to give me a nod of acknowledgment. We hadn't seen each other in years, but he knew exactly who I was. When he mouthed my name, "Bernardine" I lowered my head again and covered my mouth with a tissue to try and hide another sudden burst of grief.

Baby Alice, who sat next to me, reached over and laid her hand firmly on my arm as if I was a child she was trying to comfort and quiet. I did my best to calm down, but words from an old Peggy Lee song clanging in my head only made me cry harder: *Is That All There Is?*

When I'd heard that song as a teenager, I was horrified at the idea that life could be so fleeting, so meaningless. However, as I sat staring at my father's casket, I wondered if Miss Lee was right. Is that all there is? Is that all the time we get with Bernard Hayes—me, Uncle George, and others, I'm sure, who had unfinished emotional business with the man, who were waiting to have that heart to heart, that hug, that quiet moment with him? I waited too long. Now my father was gone, and I was sick. Can there be no healing between us now? Is that all there is?

Baby Alice touched my arm again, signaling that I should look toward the pulpit. My Mother's younger sister, Lorraine was taking a seat at the piano. I looked down at the program and realized that I'd been so lost in my thoughts I'd heard little of the minister's message or the eulogy. Aunt Lorraine was preparing to play the recessional, "When We All Get to Heaven."

Oh, boy, I thought. More tears will surely flow now. "When We All Get to Heaven" is one of those old-time gospel tunes designed to stir the soul. While Aunt Lorraine could play any kind of music, from classical to soul, she was steeped in the gospel tradition. She'd been a church pianist for decades and was known for bringing the most sedate congregation to its feet. Lorraine Grady knew exactly which tempo, chords, and progressions would have the most emotional impact on her listeners and wasn't afraid to employ them. At Daddy's service, Aunt Lorraine didn't disappoint. Almost everyone in the church recognized the song as soon as her fingers began to fly up and down the piano keys. Daddy hadn't spent much time in church, and I had no idea where he was going in the afterlife, but that afternoon, the congregation at Tindley, including me, tried their best to sing him into heaven. After a few lines, everyone was singing, clapping, and swaying to the music: *When we all get to heaven, what a day of rejoicing that will be....*

Out of the corner of my eye, I saw my brother Jerry help my mother from her seat and toward the church door. She was leaning on his arm, crying softly and still whispering my father's name. Since Daddy's death, we'd all worried about Mommy's emotional state. She had been known to pass out at funerals. She had heart failure and stayed in the hospital for a month after I got pregnant and left home. Now she was burying her husband of fifty-four years.

"Lord," I prayed to a God I wasn't sure was listening, "please let her be okay."

Aunt Lorraine was on the third verse of "When We All Get to Heaven" and the mourners sang more fervently than ever. In a moment of levity, I thought, *if these folks are trying to sing Daddy into heaven, we might be here all day.*

My moment of levity didn't last long. The pallbearers, Rob and several of his cousins walked to the front of the church to escort Daddy's casket out to the hearse. They were a beautiful rainbow of young men in their dark suits; limbs from Daddy's tree; all sharp as tacks and clean as the board of health. On another day, any one of them could be mistaken for a GQ model, but today they were grief-stricken grandchildren burying their grandfather. They adored and respected "Grandpop." He was hard on them all from time to time, but nowhere near as hard as he'd been on his own children. Seeing my son Robert so torn up brought fresh tears to my eyes. I felt sorry for my only child. He still knew nothing about my illness and had no idea of the new sadness that was waiting for him.

I don't remember the ride to the Holy Sepulcher Cemetery where Daddy was buried. I'm sure I rode in the undertaker's big black car reserved for immediate family and stood silently beside the graveside with my siblings. I may have even placed a flower on top of Daddy's casket. I know for certain, however, that Mommy wasn't at the burial. My brother took her home right from the church. Later she would explain, "I just couldn't see them put my husband in the cold ground."

∼

AFTER THE BURIAL, a crowd gathered back at my parents' house for a traditional repast. I felt Daddy's absence as soon as I stepped from the front porch into the living room. This had been Daddy's house. He'd worked years to move his family from 1437 Montrose Street—a tiny, ragged, South Philly row house, where he and his wife had to sleep in the living room, to 1426 Somerville Avenue, a roomy six-bedroom in the Logan neighborhood on the other side of town. Both the house and the neighborhood had deteriorated a bit since Daddy had brought his family here two decades ago. But the house on Somerville had been my father's pride and joy, and nothing happened here without his knowledge or consent. I looked at the people sitting comfortably on Daddy's furniture and at his dining room table, waiting to eat his food. Some were relatives, some were friends of the family, and some were folks from Tindley Temple. Mommy had had it for the day and had gone up to bed.

Daddy was gone, but the feast on the dining room table looked like his handiwork: fried chicken, pork chops, sweet potatoes swimming in butter, lettuce and tomato salad covered in mayonnaise, barbeque ribs, string beans with pork seasoning, potato salad, fried whiting, rice and gravy, rolls, fruit punch and more. I knew my youngest sister Linda prepared every dish. She had sharpened her cooking skills under Daddy's tutelage. *What's the difference between me and Linda,* I wondered. Daddy and I could never work together on anything.

"Could someone please bless the food so we can eat?" Linda called from the kitchen. I heard a murmur of appreciation roll up from the guests who'd been milling around in the dining room, devouring the spread with their eyes. Baby Alice's son, Albert, a youth leader in his Seventh Day Adventist church, raised his voice above the chatter.

I loved to hear my nephew Albert appeal to God. He always seemed so sincere, like he was simply asking a favor of a friend. Besides, he was such a beautiful physical specimen of our family. I concentrated deeply as he asked God to "mend our broken hearts on this sad day…and bless the food we needed at this time for the nourishment of our bodies," a perfect prayer for the occasion.

I quickly moved out of the way so that others, surging towards the table like a ravenous mob, could get closer to the food. At past family gatherings, I'd stuff myself with potato salad and fried whiting, right along with the other guests. But today, I wasn't hungry. Of course, my body could have been reacting to the stress of Daddy's illness, sudden death, and the morning's funeral. But also, I rarely ate heavy food like that anymore. Years ago, I'd cut pork and red meat from my diet, but over the past several months in my desperate fight with FSGS, I'd significantly reduced the amount of fried, highly salted, sugary, and fatty foods that I ate. Suddenly, I started to feel ill. I found a chair in the corner of the room where I could see everyone on the first floor of my parents' house. As I surveyed the people lifting heaping forkfuls of food into their mouths, I realized that almost every person I laid eyes on was overweight—many by more than a few pounds. *No wonder so many of us are sick or dropping dead early. We eat too damn much of all the wrong foods.*

Soon, I was well into an internal rant about how my kidney disease was probably a result of being raised on the kind of food now laid out in front of me. A hand on my shoulder pulled me back to reality. My big sister, Baby Alice. I'd know that touch anywhere. I turned around. I hadn't seen her smile in a long time.

"Hi, B. Are you okay?"

When my sister Baby Alice smiles, dimples seem to devour her cheeks, and her eyes sparkle like two stars dropped from heaven. As she stood behind my chair, I looked up at her trying to remember the first time I saw her face. Was I an infant lying in my crib when she looked down at me? But in this brief moment, memories of my sister flashed across my mind one after the other as if I was looking through one of those viewfinders she and I used to play with as kids: ten-year-old Baby Alice grinning and wearing a green and white "Lady and the Tramp" dress complete with matching pocketbook, her hair combed into three fat plaits, each tied with white ribbons; Baby Alice at thirteen smiling and ladylike with her hair pressed and curled, wearing what was likely her first grown-up dress—a yellow, flowered "fit and flair." Baby Alice as we laughed and talked, walking together to the bookmobile after school, to Rittenhouse Square on a Sunday afternoon, or the Italian Market for food shopping on Saturdays. She was always there, and I had worshiped her—everything about her.

I wanted to be just like her—shapely, and always fashionable and sophisticated to my still-young eyes. I remember sneaking out of the house wearing to school the clothes my big sister bought to wear to work, or church, or on dates. I'm sure I looked ridiculous. And then she was gone. Baby Alice got married in 1968 at twenty-one, to the boy who took her to senior prom. I felt like she left me. We drifted apart, geographically and in the lives we'd chosen. She'd spent the last thirty years as a wife and mother, living in the suburban town of Highland, New York and working part-time so she could be home when her children came in from school. I, on the other hand, was a twice-divorced, single parent with a professional career. My Robert was a latch-key kid.

"B, are you okay?" Baby Alice asked, touching my shoulder again. "Where did you go? What's the matter with you?"

This time when I looked at my sister she wasn't smiling. She looked worried—and there was something else I realized: I hadn't truly looked at my sister Alice in a long time. The young, model-thin, chic big sister from my girlhood was gone. She'd gotten older and heavier. But who was I to judge anyone? I certainly didn't look the same as I did thirty years ago.

"B" Alice hissed. "Are you okay?"

"Yes, I'm sorry. I was lost in thought. I'm okay, just a bit tired. How are you, Sister? Been a long day, right?"

"Yes, Lord," Baby Alice said keeping her eyes trained on my face. "Long day. Did you see Uncle George crying his eyes out? He was torn up! I feel sorry for him, but it's too late now. He and Daddy spent their whole lives fighting. Now Daddy's gone and there's nothing Uncle George can do about it," she said shaking her head.

"Nope," I said softly.

"Bernardine, what's wrong with you?" she asked, sounding exasperated. "You don't look well."

"Are you saying I look bad?" I asked defensively. No matter what was going on inside my body, I still had my vanity.

Alice let go of a long breath and rolled her eyes.

"No, I'm not saying you look bad, B, but what's wrong with your eyes? Why do you have such dark bags under your eyes? Are you ill?"

All I could do was stare at my sister. The entire English language deserted me and left me tongue-tied. What's more, I still had tears left in my eyes from the morning's service. If I let my sister get to me, tears would surely start to fall again. Why couldn't she leave me alone? Did she think I was blind? I knew I had bags under my eyes. Of course, she would notice. People all around us laughed and talked like they were at a party, gobbling Linda's food. None of them seemed to notice the mini drama playing out between me and my sister. Alice and I were on the sofa in the living room staring at each other—she, waiting for an answer to her question; me, silently pleading with her to let things be.

I blinked first. "Sis," I said, as I lowered my eyes and sighed, "I'm very tired. I've got a lot going on."

But my explanation wasn't enough for Baby Alice. She kept her eyes on me with a look that said, "Go on, keep talking."

I glanced up at her again. Damn! Baby Alice looked just like our mother, Alice—same round face, full cheeks, lively brown eyes. She was acting like she was my mother too. I couldn't lie to that face and tell her nothing was wrong. I also didn't have the energy to talk about FSGS right then. I didn't even have the energy to pronounce the full name of the disease.

"Look, Sis," I said, with a tinge of capitulation in my voice. "There's something I want to talk with you about. When are you leaving to go home? Can you meet me at the Reading Terminal tomorrow morning?" The Terminal was one of my favorite places in the world. Maybe the familiar surroundings would give me the courage to tell her my secret.

Alice narrowed her eyes and searched my face. I could tell she wanted to know right then what I wanted to tell her tomorrow. Thank goodness she decided not to push.

"Okay, Sis," she said again, this time more affirmatively. "I can wait until tomorrow. What time should we meet? I'll probably stay here with Mommy until Sunday. I'll get Linda or Brother Jerry to drive me downtown in the morning."

"What about around 10:00?" I suggested, thinking that after this grueling day, I didn't want to wake up too early.

"The Terminal will be crowded," I said, but before I could finish my sentence Baby Alice interrupted me.

"Don't worry, we'll find each other," she answered.

∼

BY 10:00 THE NEXT MORNING at the Reading Terminal Market, the chicken was already barbequing at Dienner's Amish Place; ducks were turning on the spit at San Kee, my favorite noodle house, and beans had been roasting for hours at Old City Coffee. The mingling aromas I identified as barbeque sauce, ginger, five-spice, and coffee all smelled beautifully familiar. But this wasn't going to be one of my usual Saturdays at the Terminal. Whether I liked it or not, I had a mission to accomplish.

I warily headed over to the main seating area, prepared to start searching for my sister. Baby Alice was right. We had no trouble finding each other. It was still early. Baby Alice had secured one of the prime tables at the end of the main seating area. Thankfully, we wouldn't be so hemmed in by the crowds and could talk in private. She looked happy and waved when she saw me. I hated the idea of making her sad with my news.

"Hey, Sis," I said with exaggerated enthusiasm. I was nervous.

"Hi, Bernardine," Baby Alice answered. She used my full name more than anyone else in the family. I took a deep breath and tried to calm myself. Baby Alice stood up and hugged me tightly.

"Do you want to get something to eat or drink?" she asked. Her cup of tea was already sitting on the table.

"No, no, I'm fine," I said as I settled into a chair directly across from her. I wanted to see the first look on her face when I told her my news. "I had coffee before I left my house."

"Coffee!" she said with an exaggerated frown on her face. "I didn't know you drank coffee. We didn't have coffee in the house when we were growing up. We always drank tea," she said, sounding as if I'd broken a family rule by drinking coffee.

"I know, I know," I said. "I still love tea and drink it all the time. I started drinking coffee when I lived in Minnesota. In restaurants, waiters sit a big pot of coffee on the table along with a pitcher of water."

"Okay," she said, shrugging as if accepting that she couldn't do anything about my coffee habit. "What did you want to talk with me about?"

Right then, I wished I had a cup of coffee or even tea in my hand, anything to hold on to, anything that might stop my hands from shaking so visibly. But there was nothing I could do except open my mouth and let the words come out—but not too loudly. The Market was filling up and people were sitting at one of the tables next to ours.

"I have kidney disease and will probably need a transplant," I blurted out. I could hardly believe the words I'd just said.

Baby Alice stared at me. She seemed to not react to my words. I even wondered if she heard what I said. Then my sister lowered her head. I think she was praying. When she lifted her eyes, I saw her sorrow.

"Oh B," she said. "I'm so sorry." Baby Alice reached across the table, took my hand, and repeated herself. "When did you find out about this? What's the doctor saying?"

I took a deep breath and started at the beginning, with that day in 1984, fifteen years ago, when a doctor told me I had excess protein in my urine—a possible sign of kidney disease.

"You can imagine how I felt," I said to Alice. "I thought the doctor was over-reacting—being extra careful. As far as I know, kidney disease doesn't run in our family."

Alice listened, shaking her head in empathy.

"Besides, Sis," I continued. "1984 was an awful year in my life. I don't know if you remember that I was still living in Minnesota. My marriage to Alexs was breaking up, and I was about to lose my job. On top of all that, I had to deal with this bad health news."

Baby Alice never took her eyes off me as I described that

time in my life. Most of this information was news to her. I wondered if she was thinking the same thing I was. *Damn, I wish I'd kept in better touch with my sister.* But there was nothing either of us could do about that now.

I went on to tell her about my shock at learning the FSGS diagnosis from the specialist, and my relief when I was told at the Mayo Clinic that the disease might never progress.

"And it didn't progress, Alice. Not for many years."

"You shouldn't have gone through all this by yourself, B," Alice finally said, pursing her lips and shaking her head at me. "You should have called me."

What could I say? I didn't call. My sister knew as well as I did that we hadn't stayed in touch, even though we couldn't exactly explain why. Besides, I couldn't remember the last time I asked one of my siblings for help.

"Where do things stand now?" Alice asked.

"Well, my doctor says my kidney function is diminishing. He says by the end of the year, I'll probably need dialysis or a transplant and that I should be thinking about potential kidney donors."

A long silence settled in between us as my sister absorbed that news.

"Dialysis is awful, B," Alice said.

I flinched. With everything I was facing, dialysis was what I feared most.

People were now sitting on either side of us. Someone was eating a cheesesteak with fried onions. I hadn't eaten beef in years, but that steak smelled good. Alice recognized the smell too and gave me a sly look. As a Seventh Day Adventist, she didn't eat meat now at all, but we'd grown up on those delicious sandwiches. "Listen," Alice said. I immediately leaned toward her so I could hear her above the growing din. "Everything is going to be okay. We're going to trust in the Lord, and everything is going to be okay."

I found myself wishing I had her faith.

"Come up to Mommy's tomorrow. I'm sure Linda and Judy will be there. I'm not sure about Brother Jerry, he may be going back to New York today. We'll talk about this as a family and figure things out. You can't go through this alone."

I repeated my sister's words in my head. *We'll talk through this as a family*—a family I sometimes didn't feel part of.

I nodded but insisted on one condition.

"I don't want to tell Mommy yet. I can't put this on her now."

"I know, I know," Alice said. "We'll worry about Mommy later. Right now, we'll worry about you." Alice paused for a moment as if carefully considering her next words, then she completed her thought.

"And if you need a kidney, we'll talk about that tomorrow too."

I groaned in dismay. After years of keeping my distance from my family, now I have to tell my siblings my deepest secrets. In the past two days, we'd put Daddy into the ground, and I'd told Alice the secret I'd kept for fifteen years. Things were spinning out of my control. But I was out of choices.

Chapter Four:
EVERYTHING'S GOING TO BE OKAY

Once I told Baby Alice I needed a kidney, she went into full "big sister" mode. The next day she corralled me and my siblings into the back bedroom at Mommy's house and closed the door behind us.

"Go ahead, B, tell them," she commanded. Suddenly, the sisterly closeness I'd been feeling toward Alice over the past few days began to evaporate. I resented her bossiness. Do I have to tell everyone my business? The answer was obvious. Yes, I did. Besides, I couldn't remember the last time I needed my family so much. I looked around the bedroom at my siblings. Judith, or Judy, who was two years younger than me, sat beside me at the foot of the bed. Judy had been the gentle one among my siblings, the quietest one. During our adolescence, when I was so busy trying to keep up with my older sister Alice, I hadn't paid her much attention. Now, Judy seemed to loom over me, waiting to hear my secret. Linda, the youngest of the Hayes girls, sat at the head of the bed with her arms tightly folded across her chest. She was the prettiest of the Hayes sisters in my opinion and feisty from birth. Now the look on her face read, *just get on with it and tell me what's going on.* Brother Jerry, the youngest in the family, had already left to go back home to New York.

I could feel Baby Alice's eyes on me. There was no way I could get out of that room without spilling the beans. One more time, I launched into my tale of woe, finishing with, "I'll need a kidney soon."

Once I said those words, I breathed a loud sigh and glanced at Baby Alice.

There, I told them, my look said.

Baby Alice nodded her approval. For a few seconds, no one moved or said a word. Finally, my sister Judy whispered, "Wow." Then there was silence again.

"Is this disease hereditary?" Linda asked finally, her voice cracking a little by the time she got to the end of the question. "Do we all need to get our urine tested for protein?"

I'd asked my doctors the same question many times and still wasn't clear. I didn't want to send everyone into a panic.

"Lin, I don't understand everything about FSGS. The doctors don't either. Believe me, I've asked a lot of questions. My doctor, a nephrologist who specializes in kidney disease, tells me they don't know exactly why people develop FSGS. Many people who get the disease also have diabetes, lupus, or high blood pressure, but others don't. I didn't have high blood pressure when I was first diagnosed, but now I'm on medication for it."

I stopped talking for a moment, surprised at the tears stinging behind my eyelids. Remembering the day Dr. Frankel told me I had high blood pressure still made me sad. Then I continued my explanation.

"Just because I have FSGS, doesn't mean any of you do or will. Daddy was diabetic but he didn't have this disease, and Mommy doesn't either. Just my luck," I laughed. No one laughed with me.

"One important thing is true, though," I continued, "FSGS

is prevalent among African Americans and other Black and brown people. So you probably should have the kidney function test anyway."

"Have you told Robby yet?" Linda asked.

I hung my head and looked at the floor. Leave it to my feisty little sister, Linda, to ask the tough questions. I felt ashamed that I hadn't told Robert about my disease. I couldn't bear to. No matter the difficulties Rob and I had from time to time, I knew that I was the one person he truly depended on.

"I haven't," I said hesitantly. "I don't want to scare him, but I guess I'll have to tell him soon."

I was exhausted. I wanted to stop talking. I'd said all I could say. The room smelled sour and felt stuffy with sweat and fear. The fear was probably my own.

"Listen," Alice said firmly, as her three younger sisters turned to face her. "Yes, we should all get tested for protein in our urine. In fact, at some point, we should tell our kids about this disease, so they get tested too. But I don't want Mommy knowing about this until we've figured out what we're going to do about B."

We all nodded our heads yes. Deep inside though, I was having a very different conversation with myself. I couldn't imagine ever telling Mommy that I had kidney disease. Mommy went into the hospital with heart failure after I told her I was pregnant, and I still felt responsible.

"And while we're getting tested for the disease, we might as well get tested to see who's compatible with B. One of us is going to have to be her donor. We can't let her go on dialysis. Dialysis is awful and she could be waiting years for a kidney."

I looked at my other two sisters to see how they were taking to Alice's directive. Judy, the quiet one, began to talk.

"What's wrong with dialysis?" she asked. "Our friend Grayland from church has been on dialysis for years, and he's doing okay."

I couldn't believe my ears. Sweet Judy had summed up the cold reality of my situation. I was fucked! I'd wrestled with the fact that I had kidney disease. The idea of a transplant—having someone else's kidney sewn into my body—freaked me out. But Judy had put her finger right on the sore spot. If I didn't get a transplant, I could be tied to a machine for the rest of my life. Hellfire and brimstone couldn't be worse as far as I was concerned. I wondered if Judy was telling me that I was no better than other people? Was she telling me that I wasn't entitled to anyone else's kidney? Maybe she was right.

"Just wait a minute," Alice interjected. "We're getting ahead of ourselves. Why don't we all get tested and see what's what? Can you arrange that appointment, B, and let us know what to do?"

Judy, Linda, and I all nodded obediently. Baby Alice let out a long sigh of relief. The meeting was over, and she'd gotten what she wanted—the unity among the sisters that Daddy would have approved of. We'd still have to wait and see what Brother Jerry had to say.

Alice hugged each of us. She'd earned her big sister stripes that day. How could I be angry with her? When she put her arms around me, whispering that everything was going to be okay, I wasn't sure I agreed, but I hugged her back.

I opened the door to the bedroom and a wave of fresh air poured in. I looked down the dark hallway and saw that Mommy's door was still closed. I could feel Daddy's absence. There's no way we all could have been in that room with the door closed for an hour without Daddy coming in and demanding, "What y'all doing in here?"

I TRIED TO BELIEVE Baby Alice… that everything was going to be okay. I repeated her words like a mantra. When I next saw Dr. Rudnick, in June, 1999, I'd lost more kidney function—my creatinine level was 6.2. The Vasotec he'd prescribed for my blood pressure wasn't working as well as we'd hoped. Rudnick had originally described the pill as "a miracle drug," so of course, I'd expected miracles. Initially, the Vasotec had lowered my pressure and reduced the amount of protein in my urine. However, the good results didn't last long. FSGS was determined to have its way with my body.

"FSGS is a wretched disease," Rudnick said, sounding as if he were talking about an old foe he'd battled many times. "I thought the Vasotec would buy us more time." He began to scribble out new prescriptions on his pad. "Have you started looking for donors yet?" he asked.

"I talked with my family and my three sisters are going to be tested."

"You don't sound very excited," he said dryly. "Your three sisters? That's great news. I have dialysis patients that would kill for just one donor let alone three sisters. All three sisters could be good matches for you. You're very fortunate."

Rudnick put down his pen and looked directly into my face. He didn't seem annoyed, but concerned and sympathetic.

"Ms. Watson, I know this is a lot to take in. I'm sorry you must go through this but believe me, you are one of the lucky ones. You don't have an underlying condition like diabetes or lupus, and you're a good candidate for a kidney transplant. You have good insurance, you have the kind of family support we like to see, and you have potential donors. I'd recommend that you and your sisters go over to the transplant clinic at the University of Pennsylvania and get tested for compatibility. Do it soon! If you have a donor who's tested, and ready by the time you need the kidney, you may never have to be on dialysis. I told you before that dialysis can be extremely hard on the body. I can get you an appointment at Penn. Let me know when you're ready to get started."

However, no matter Rudnick's warnings, I wasn't ready to start planning for a transplant. 1999 had already laid me low and June wasn't even over yet. That July, my birthday month, I took all four weeks of my vacation. My goal was to try not to think too much about my failing kidneys. Except for a bit of fatigue which by now was my normal state, I didn't feel bad. I'd take the time for myself. Who knew what the future held?

During this month-long respite, I slept late, took afternoon naps, and became a regular at Toppers, a spa in my neighborhood—treating myself to manicures, pedicures, facials, and massages. I also got involved in an on-again, off-again relationship with a beautiful, talented, troubled man—a jazz drummer and former heroin addict, who'd kicked his drug habit but not all his "druggy" behaviors. We met at a party, and I don't think we'd have gotten past "hello" if I'd been in a different state of mind. When we were "on" we were magic—slow dancing in the middle of my living room floor, listening to Miles Davis or Joe Henderson blow late into the dark sky outside my bedroom window, or to Shirley Horn meandering through a lovely ballad.

When we were "off" though, we were very off, and I'd swear I'd never see him again…until I did. He helped me forget for a while.

Still, no matter how hard I tried to forget, there was always something to remind me about the FSGS that was destroying my kidneys and my life: the amber-colored pill bottles on my kitchen counter and the teas, potions, and vitamins in my kitchen cabinet that I obtained from the herbalist I saw regularly. Based on my test results, there wasn't one ounce of evidence these "alternative medicines" were doing me any good. For all I knew, they were harming me. Still, every day, I drank ginseng and dandelion tea and took the milk thistle and sage capsules. Dr. Rudnick would have had a fit if he knew I was taking the stuff. He scoffed at anything other than traditional medicine.

On Labor Day, my musician friend and I had a picnic in a secluded spot in Fairmount Park. All afternoon we lay close to each other on the grass and listened to the be-bop and hard-bop of Bud Powell and Hank Mobley on a big 1980's boom box that still had great sound. I was happy that day, but happiness didn't stick around.

On September 8th, the Wednesday after Labor Day, I kept my scheduled appointment with Dr. Rudnick. He'd moved from Graduate Hospital at 18th and Lombard in downtown to Presbyterian, or Presby as the locals called it, at 39th and Filbert in West Philly. I hoped a summer of relative relaxation and male company had been good for me. Maybe Rudnick would tell me something good.

"Hello, Ms. Watson," he said in his usual monotone when I walked into the examination room. "Your creatinine is up," he said. His words hung in the air like a bad odor. "Have you talked to your sisters again?"

"Not yet." I responded in a voice so even and calm that I surprised my own ears. "But I will as soon as I get home."

Rudnick reached into the top pocket of his white coat and pulled a business card from behind his stethoscope.

"Call Susan Kirkland," he said. "She's a nurse and the transplant coordinator at Penn. Tell her I told you to call. She'll help you and your sisters with the testing." Dr. Rudnick then slapped his hands against his thighs and stood up, telling me without saying a word that we were done. My summer break was over. Dr. Rudnick had predicted that I would need a transplant or dialysis by the end of 1999. Here we were in September, and he was sending me and my sisters over to Penn for a transplant evaluation. I had no choice but to face the cool fall winds blowing in my direction.

I called each of my sisters that afternoon to tell them the latest news and make sure they were still willing to be tested. How could I blame any one of them if they had changed their minds? I also called the Penn Transplant Center and made an appointment for me and my sisters with Nurse Kirkland. I decided to leave my brother Jerry out of things for the time being.

Judy wasn't able to make the appointment, but within a few weeks, Alice, Linda, and I were in the basement of the main building of the University of Penn hospital. The sign on the door read: Transplant Institute: Kidney, Liver, Pancreas and Lung Clinic. I could see through the window that the waiting room was packed with people, mostly White. Where were all the Black people? Every doctor I'd seen told me that kidney disease affected more Black people than any other group. Why weren't we in the transplant clinic?

My sisters and I stood for a moment at the clinic door looking at each other. *If anybody wants to change their mind, now is the time*, I thought. Alice must have read my mind.

"We might as well go in," she said. When I reached the front desk, a young man looked up and asked kindly, "What clinic are you here for?"

"Kidney," I whispered as if I didn't want anyone to hear me. Why the hell was I whispering? Almost everybody in this room was here to see about replacing one body part or another.

"Sign in here," the man said, pointing to the sheet that said "KIDNEY" across the top in big red letters. Our appointment was at 9:00. It was 8:59. Already we were number seven.

We sat in the waiting room for over an hour—making quiet small talk, flipping through magazines, and waiting. I couldn't remember the last time the three of us were together outside of Mommy and Daddy's house. We hadn't remained close over the years, but sitting in the waiting room, a calm familiarity settled over us. We were sisters, three of the Hayes girls, and not even time could change that.

I glanced around the waiting room casually trying not to stare at people but wondering about the stories behind their faces. Who was ailing and who was well? Who were the potential donors and who would be the recipients? Most of the people in the room looked normal. Others were visibly ill—like the woman sitting directly across from me wearing a mask over her nose and mouth, or the guy with the greenish cast to his skin. As I spent more time in the transplant clinic, I learned that greenish skin could mean a critical case of liver disease. I looked over at my sisters.

"I hope it's not too much longer," I mouthed. Alice had driven down from New York the day before for this appointment, and Lin had taken time from work. I hated for them to have to sit here all day.

"Bernardine Watson."

Hallelujah! A chubby brown woman standing at the front desk was calling my name. She called out my name again before I could pop out of my chair.

"Here I am, here I am," I said loudly as I started to make my way across the room.

I looked back at my sisters and made an exaggerated happy face. Everyone still sitting and waiting seemed to watch me enviously as I hurried up to the desk.

"Bernardine Watson," I announced to the woman, surprised at how heavily I was breathing. I felt winded even though I'd only walked a few feet. Maybe I was nervous. Or maybe the FSGS was now affecting my lungs. Honestly, I could no longer trust my body.

"How are you today?" the woman said warmly. "I'm Susan Kirkland, the transplant coordinator. Are your sisters here?"

"I'm well as I can be, thank you. My sisters are sitting right over there." I pointed to Linda and Alice, surprised at how proud I felt to have them with me.

"Well, let's get them over here," Kirkland said enthusiastically, beckoning vigorously to my sisters to come across the room. Suddenly, all eyes in the room seemed to be on the Hayes girls.

"Please," said Kirkland politely. "Come with me." She made a grand sweep toward a hallway with her right arm, while holding my medical file and some pamphlets in her left. We followed her into a small room.

"Sit down, please," she said, pointing to a few folding chairs scattered about. "I think we should be able to grab this space for a while without being interrupted. To say that space is at a premium around here would definitely be an understatement," she said, laughing.

Kirkland was pretty in a plain way, the kind of woman with basic good looks—smooth skin, pleasant features, a thick, healthy head of hair—but who did nothing to fix herself up. No make-up, her natural hair pulled back in an Afro puff, and her clothes unremarkable. She wore a simple skirt and blouse under her white lab coat.

"Now, tell me who is who," Kirkland continued, laying the files down on a table and picking up a yellow legal pad and pen. "Give me your birthdays also," she said, scribbling all the while.

"Okay," she said, laying down her pen. "Bernardine, Alice, Linda. I'll try to remember. Please call me Susan. I'm the transplant coordinator for the kidney and pancreas program. My job is to make sure that anyone who comes to our program has an exceptional experience, whether you are a potential donor or recipient and whether you end up taking part in our program or not. I must say I'm especially glad to meet all of you. You all are a sight for sore eyes."

Ha. I thought Mommy was the only one who used the phrase, "a sight for sore eyes." I was also curious about why she was especially glad to see us. Were we special? Susan must have seen the curiosity on my face and started talking again.

"You have to understand," she said, lowering her voice even though the office door was closed. "We don't see as many Black people in transplant clinic as we'd like—recipients or donors, let alone three sisters."

"Why is that?" I asked.

"Well," Susan said, still speaking softly, "transplantation is a complicated business. Getting a kidney transplant or a transplant of any kind, for that matter, requires time and resources, assets that everybody doesn't have in abundance. I can give you more information about this issue at another time if you're interested. Right now, I need you ladies to fill out some paperwork. Ok? Wait here, I'll be right back," she said. Before she opened the door, Susan turned, looked back at me, and said, "Ms. Watson, you have an abundance of resources. In the transplant world, you're a rich woman."

A week later Baby Alice called with news. "We're all a match," she said. "You, me, and Linda—that's what the tissue and blood test showed."

I was speechless but remembered what Dr. Rudnick said. We were sisters with the same parents. Still, I was so tongue-tied that I couldn't talk. Finally, I was able to get a few words out.

"How do you know this?" I asked. "I haven't heard a word."

"Confidentiality. They'll only give test results to the person who took the test. Linda and I got separate calls. We'll have to do some further testing, but it looks like either of us can give you a kidney."

Baby Alice remained silent for the next few seconds, Finally, she said, "I'll do it. I'll be your donor, B."

I knew my sister was serious. She was speaking in her *I dare you to try and talk me out of this* tone—a tone I knew well. Baby Alice meant business. I could see her on the other end of the line— the telephone cradled between her shoulder and ear, both hands on her hips, her eyes defiant.

"Lin and I have already talked about it. Judy is still willing to be tested, but I'm the oldest, and I have the time, I'm not working right now."

What was I supposed to say? I couldn't think of a damn thing. "Thank you" seemed such a small, inadequate response to give to someone who offers you a body part.

"Alice," I began, but my sister stopped me.

"Look, B," she said, "You don't have to say a word. It's going to be okay. If I didn't believe in God, I wouldn't be able to let them take a kidney out of my body. But I do. I believe God will take care of both of us and bring us right on through."

I closed my eyes and tried to name the emotions coursing through my body: gratitude, relief, and of course, fear—my constant companion.

My kidney function deteriorated rapidly over the next few months. When I saw Dr. Rudnick in early December, he was clearly concerned.

"Your creatinine level is over 10," he said, looking down at me over his wire-frame glasses. "This means you have very little kidney function left. How are you feeling, Ms. Watson?"

Honestly, since I'd seen Dr. Rudnick in September, I'd been tired and sluggish. Now, the bags under my eyes looked even darker. I hated to look in the mirror. Still, I didn't want to admit how exhausted I felt.

"I'm okay," I answered. Rudnick stared at me and frowned. "Ms. Watson, the body can sometimes keep going on very little kidney function, but we're going to have to get you transplanted or on dialysis within the next month or so. Where's your sister with the testing?"

Dialysis. The word scared me to death. In my mind, dialysis equaled death.

"Dr Rudnick," I said, panicking. "I thought I could get a transplant before I needed to go on dialysis. Isn't that what you said?"

I could hear the words tumbling out of my mouth. I wondered if he knew how terrified I was.

Rudnick began speaking very slowly and clearly as if I was a little daft and he had to make sure his words sunk into my thick skull.

"No, Ms. Watson. That's not what I said. What I said is that you might not have to spend any time on dialysis if we can get you transplanted before your kidney function deteriorates too much. But your creatinine level is rising faster than I expected. Before we can seriously talk about transplant, we still need a few test results from you, and I need to talk to the folks at Penn about the transplant schedule. What about your sister? Where is she in the testing process?"

I'd heard Dr. Rudnick when he asked that question the first time. I didn't know the answer. I knew Alice had been working with the coordinator at Penn Transplant to complete the necessary tests, but I didn't know where things stood. I also knew that the list of pre-transplant tests and doctors' visits my sister needed to complete was formidable—heart studies, kidney function tests, chest X-rays, a gynecological exam, plus a psychological evaluation. Even though I, too, wanted to know where Alice was with the testing, I hadn't called her in weeks. I felt bad enough asking her for a kidney. Now I didn't want to pressure her about the testing.

When I looked up at the doctor, he was standing over me with his arms folded, waiting for my response. I took a deep breath. "I don't know where things stand, doctor. I'll call my sister today and find out."

Dr. Rudnick and I had been in a tiny examination room with the door closed for about ten minutes. The air was starting to feel hot and thick. Rudnick reached for the blood pressure cup to slip around my arm. I braced myself to see a high blood pressure reading. This was not a good time to have my pressure taken. I was too agitated.

"150/90, Ms. Watson," Rudnick said frowning "Too high. I'll take it again before you leave. Unbutton your shirt a bit please."

I tried to breathe normally as Rudnick listened to my heart.

TRANSPLANT: A MEMOIR

"Your heart sounds good," he said, shaking his head affirmatively.

Next, he felt my ankles and shook his head "yes" again. Apparently, they weren't too swollen. I let out a sigh of relief about my good heart and my relatively slim ankles. At least there was some good news from this exam.

Before I left his office, Dr. Rudnick asked about my sister, Alice, again. "Please find out where things stand with your sister. If I remember, she's up in the New York area, right? Let me know if she needs any help getting these tests completed up there. I'll make some calls if that will speed things up. I'll also check with Roy Bloom's office over at Penn Transplant to see what the transplant schedule looks like for early next year. In the meantime, make an appointment to come back and see me right after the holidays. We should know more by then. But if you start to feel sick—short of breath, dizzy, faint, call me right away. We'll talk soon, okay?"

I shook my head meekly. I couldn't believe that Dr. Rudnick and my sister Baby Alice held my life in their hands.

～

THE CHRISTMAS HOLIDAYS are one of my favorite times of the year. I love decorating, cooking, and merry-making and have been known to throw a great holiday party myself. Usually, I took time from work at the end of the year, so I could properly partake in all the festivities. However, as I sat in Rudnick's office pondering what the next several months of my life might bring, I decided that today would be my last day of work until who knew when. *Sometime in the next few months, I will have a kidney transplant.* I repeated that reality to myself. I needed time to prepare mentally and physically. Everything else had to come second—even my job. I had more than enough sick leave, and I was sure I'd qualify for short-term disability or something like that. My boss would have to understand, and if he didn't…well, I'd face that too, if necessary. I had to take care of myself.

On the surface, the holidays of 1999 were much like Christmases past, with decorations, gifts, and food. All my siblings and their families were present except Baby Alice and her crew, who had decided not to make the trek from New York that year. I certainly didn't blame her for staying put. Alice had begun the pre-operative testing for potential kidney donors and had her hands full.

Anyway, it was Daddy's absence that hovered over my parents' home, especially in the kitchen, where on Christmas Day, he would have been busy presiding over dinner preparations. Instead, my sisters, Linda and Judy were at the stove working mightily to replicate Daddy's well-known holiday dishes.

"We're going to do Daddy proud," Linda said adamantly, as she carefully covered each piece of whiting with seasoned flour and dropped it into a pan of hot oil on the top of the stove.

Of my siblings, only Baby Alice knew how close I was to kidney failure. I'd told my brother and other sisters that I was waiting for test results and would have more to share after the holidays. I wasn't about to spoil Christmas with bad tidings. While my sisters cooked furiously in the kitchen, my brother Jerry and I, and a few of the grandkids sat around the TV in the living room. But no matter where we were in the house, Daddy's commanding presence was clearly missing.

By four in the afternoon, the smell of a delicious Christmas dinner filled the house. Judy called to me from the kitchen.

"B, can you please start setting the table?"

I popped up immediately, happy to have something useful to do. My brother joined me in the dining room.

"Do you think Mommy will come downstairs and eat dinner with us?" I asked him.

Since Daddy's death in May, she'd started spending more and more time in her bedroom.

"I don't know," he responded. "I'll go up and get her when we're ready to bless the food." He and I both knew that if anyone could get her to come downstairs, it would be him, her baby boy, Bernard Jerome, named for my father.

I shuddered inside at the thought of having to face my mother. Would she be able to tell that I was faking my Christmas spirit? How much longer could I hide my illness from her? My January appointment with Rudnick was scheduled for the 5th. I had no idea what would happen after that.

Chapter Five:
HAPPY NEW YEAR TO ME

For all the calamity January 1, 2000, or Y2K, was supposed to bring to the world, the day passed in Philly with no more disruption than a few drunk Mummers staggering down Market Street. However, for me, the start of the new year was calamitous.

First, I had no choice but to tell Robert my secret. I hate to admit this, but I took the coward's way out and waited until January 4th to give him the news.

Robert and I were finally in a good place. He'd dropped out of college and bounced around for a while from job to job and place to place, including a year or two in Toronto, Canada. My feelings about Robert leaving school did not help our relationship. First, I was angry with him. Didn't he understand how hard I'd worked to get to a point where I could afford to send him to college? Didn't he know that a college degree would help protect him from some of the same economic struggles that I'd had to deal with? What the hell could he be thinking? Second—I also wondered about my own culpability. Where had I failed my son? Maybe my instability over the years—my two divorces and my moves from place to place, had affected Robert more than I realized. Maybe my best hadn't been good enough.

During this time, Robert sometimes kept his distance from me. However, when he landed a job he loved at the *Philadelphia Inquirer*, we could both exhale. He'd found success on his terms. Now I wondered if my shocking news would bring drama to his life that he didn't need.

I invited Robert to come by my apartment after work. My goal was to tell him about my illness and try to make him understand why I'd waited so long to let him know what I'd been going through. I still struggled with how to answer that question for myself. Why had I waited so long to tell Robert about my illness? Was it fear? Shame? Love? But this was D-Day. I was running out of time. "Robert can handle this," I told myself. He was tough like me. I raised him.

Robert didn't think there was anything unusual about my invitation. He often stopped by my place after work, whether I was home or not, to rummage through my refrigerator or just hang out and listen to music. Music was a love that he and I shared. I may have helped him cultivate his musical interests, but he had long since surpassed me in his musical knowledge and the variety of genres he listened to. The CD I selected for his visit was a compilation of music he'd made for me. I liked it primarily because Robert had given it to me.

"Sounds good up in here," Robert said cheerfully as he walked in the door and into my living room. For a moment all I could do was stare at my child. No matter what else was going on in my life, he never failed to make me feel better.

"Hey, son, how are you?" I asked, trying hard to sound calm and cool. "I like this CD. Isn't this Massive Attack?"

"Go 'head, Mom. That's right. I knew you would dig them—they have some of that old-school soul sound, right?

Robert tossed his coat and hat on the sofa. He walked into

the kitchen and hugged me with one arm while opening the refrigerator door with the other. Robert didn't live with me anymore, but at twenty-eight, he still felt entitled to the food or anything else in my house. He was right. I'd do anything in the world for my son no matter how old he was. I hugged him back. I was proud of him and glad to see him happy. I was so sorry I had to give him such bad news.

"Can I cook this turkey sausage?" he asked. "Got any bread? I feel like a sammich." We looked at each other and laughed. My dad used to talk about making himself a "sammich" when he was hungry and in a good mood. Robert sounded exactly like him.

"Sure," I said. "You know you can make anything you want. But first, I need to talk to you." I walked over to the sofa in the living room and sat down. If I didn't sit down, I was going to fall down.

"Can't I cook while we're talking?" he asked, still rooting around in the fridge.

I hesitated for a moment. Could I tell him about the kidney transplant while he makes a turkey-sausage sandwich? I didn't think so.

"No, son," I said. "I need your undivided attention."

For the first time since he'd entered my apartment, Robert looked directly into my face. I patted the spot on the sofa next to me, indicating where I wanted him to sit.

"Come," I said. And he headed around to the sofa, not once taking his eyes off me.

I knew from the experience of breaking this news to my siblings that this talk would be difficult for me. Still, I was especially at a loss with my child, my only child, my baby, the one I'd raised alone, the biggest part of my heart. He was grown now, but I was still his mama and he still depended on me.

"I need a kidney transplant," I said, as calmly as I could.

"Mom, what? What did you say?" he asked, drawing back from me as if he was afraid of whatever else might come out of my mouth.

"I need a kidney transplant, Robert. I've known for a while and I'm sorry I didn't tell you a long time ago."

"Is this why you're lying on the couch so often when I come over?"

All I could do was nod. My son and I searched each other's faces—I suppose for some clue about what to do or say next. I reached over and touched Robert's hand. I could tell from the tears in his eyes that my words were slowly sinking in.

Robert didn't ask for any details. We just sat on the sofa for a few minutes, listening to the music he'd given me. We both knew that whatever the future held, there'd be plenty of time for talking.

~

When I arrived at Dr. Rudnick's office on January 5th, he was standing in the waiting area, seeming distracted and rushed.

"Good morning, Ms. Watson. How are you?" he said as he scribbled on his prescription pad.

"I'm okay, Dr. Rudnick. You'll be glad to hear that my sister has completed most of her tests. She has a few more tests to go. The results should be over at Penn."

"Good, glad to hear that, Ms. Watson," Rudnick said, still seeming distracted.

I waited for a moment to hear what else Dr. Rudnick was going to say. I was nervous. This was the day I was supposed to find out the next steps in treating my failing kidneys.

"I'm sorry, Ms. Watson. I have an emergency and must

leave," Rudnick said as he tore a sheet from his prescription pad and handed it to me.

"Take this over to Intervention Radiology, fourth floor in the Wright Saunders Building. Also, you should make an appointment to come in and see me next week."

Rudnick then disappeared out of his office door and down the hallway. I was dumbfounded. What the hell is Intervention Radiology? I didn't even know where the Wright Saunders building was.

Once I walked out of Rudnick's office, I saw signs that I'd never noticed before pointing to "Wright Saunders." As I made my way through the winding hallways, I could feel my stomach churning and my mind racing. Intervention Radiology? Why do I have to go there? I'm not a child to be told what to do without an explanation. I thought about going home and calling Rudnick later so he could explain what was going on. I looked quickly at the paper he'd handed me but couldn't read his handwriting. However, since I'd come all the way uptown for this appointment, I might as well stay and not waste the time.

As I crossed over into the Wright Saunders building, I began to panic. Sweat dripped down the back of my sweater. I suspected why Rudnick was sending me over to Wright Saunders. This has something to do with dialysis, I thought. Intervention Radiology. Dialysis is one of the most invasive procedures there is. With each step, I grew more certain that Rudnick had arranged for me to talk with someone about dialysis. Why didn't he tell me? I stared at the elevator doors for a moment and finally pushed the up button. I decided that I might as well hear whatever the folks had to say. I already felt awful. Why not destroy the entire day?

To my eye, the fourth floor of Wright Saunders was as drab

and depressing as every other floor in Presbyterian Hospital—faded beige walls, lifeless grey floors, and unhappy people waiting on unhappy people.

"Sign in right here," a young Black woman said before I even reached her desk. "I also need your insurance card, I.D, your order, name, and date of birth."

"Bernardine Watson, 7-16-1951," I said wearily as I handed everything, including Rudnick's scribbled note.

The young woman copying down my information seemed as bored and uninterested in her job as I was in being at the hospital that day. I looked at her vacant face as she pushed a clipboard in my direction. She was young—maybe in her 20's—and beautiful. Her skin was the color of a Bosc pear, and her eyes were…green? Light brown? I wondered why such a beautiful young woman would be stuck behind a desk in a little cubicle looking at sick people all day. Life can be so unfair! The name tag pinned to her blue top read "Regina."

"Thank you, Regina," I said, lightly, trying to put myself and Regina in a better mood.

"You're welcome," she said, seeming surprised by our pleasant exchange.

"Have a seat and listen for your name," Regina said kindly.

I found a seat beside an older Black man, wriggled out of my coat, and sighed as I settled into the chair. Sitting around in hospital waiting rooms was becoming the story of my life.

Before I pulled out my novel, I took a good look around the waiting room. I'd been so busy grumbling about my situation and wondering about the young woman at the reception desk, I'd barely noticed the other people in the room: Black folks everywhere, not a White face to be seen. To a person they looked weary, worn out, sick, and tired. Sick and tired of being sick and tired, I thought to myself, recalling the words of Fannie Lou Hamer.

I thought back to the Transplant Center at the University of Pennsylvania where my sisters and I were the only Black people in the waiting room, and where you could barely tell the sick from the well. Here everyone looked sick. The clock on the wall said 10:00 a.m., but at least a quarter of the people in the room were slumped over and sleeping. Across the aisle from me, a woman sat in a wheelchair with a heavy green army blanket covering where her legs used to be. I couldn't remember when I'd seen this much misery in one place. I couldn't help thinking about my conversation with the nurse in the Transplant Center. "We don't see many Black people here," she said. Apparently, all the Black people were in Intervention Radiology—including me. I pulled Frank McCourt's *Angela's Ashes* out of my bag, ready to be transported to dire poverty in Limerick. Once I left college and no longer had to read the books I was assigned, I'd stopped buying books by White men. Increasingly, I wanted to support Black writers and read books that reflected my experience. Still, I'd heard McCourt interviewed on NPR and was taken with his Irish lilt and the few seductive paragraphs he'd read from his memoir. McCourt's squalid Irish Catholic childhood kept my eyes glued to the page until I heard my name called.

"Bernardine Watson." The beautiful young woman's voice was back to being as listless as when I'd entered the room an hour ago. The morning wasn't over yet and already she sounded like she'd been at her desk for the whole day. Regina needed a new job.

"Go down this hallway to the door on the left," she said. I nodded as I passed her desk. A nurse in blue medical scrubs was waiting for me on the other side of the door.

"Name and date of birth?" she asked.

For heaven's sake, I thought. How many times do I have to repeat this information? But after a sigh, I answered calmly.

"My name is Theresa and I'll be assisting with your procedure this morning. Let's get your temperature and blood pressure," she said as she pointed to a chair in an examining room.

Theresa's words stopped me in my tracks.

"What procedure?" The calm in my voice had disappeared.

The woman looked at me quizzically. "You don't know why you're here?" Her voice rose with disbelief and exasperation. I responded in kind.

"Dr. Rudnick sent me here, maybe to talk with someone about dialysis. He didn't say anything about a procedure."

I began to feel dizzy. A familiar fear settled in the pit of my stomach.

The nurse looked down at the papers on her clipboard.

"I know who sent you," she said patiently. "I know Dr. Rudnick. I've been a nurse in this department for quite a while. I see his patients all the time. Your order says, 'Insert catheter, right chest, for hemodialysis.' Dr. Rudnick didn't explain this to you?" Theresa shut the examining room door and pointed me to a chair.

Am I losing my mind, I thought? Could I have forgotten this conversation with Rudnick, or not heard him correctly? No. I don't think so. I might be stressed, but I'm not crazy.

"No," I mumbled. "He didn't explain…." I let the rest of my sentence trail off. Embarrassed and angry to find myself in this situation, I couldn't finish my sentence. How could this happen? I'm a grown-ass woman, goddammit! I stared at the floor. I didn't want the nurse to see me cry.

"Look, Ms. Watson," the nurse said kindly. "You don't have to do this today if you don't want to. You seem very upset."

She paused and waited for me to respond, but I didn't say a word. My head was full of hot tears that I'd been holding in for what seemed like a lifetime. Now I was in danger of boiling over. The nurse sighed heavily.

"Ms. Watson, I don't know what happened here. I said you don't have to have this procedure today, but I'd recommend you have it. If Dr. Rudnick sent you to have a catheter inserted, you should. You need dialysis, so this is in your best interest. This seems like a shock to you, but you're going to have to do this eventually. It's up to you." She handed me a tissue.

You're going to have to do this eventually. The nurse's words echoed.

The catheter insertion was nothing less than torture—maybe because I was upset before the procedure started or maybe because catheter insertion is torture. This procedure was done with a local anesthetic, so I was awake as the radiologist pushed a plastic tube into a vein in my neck. He seemed to have no more compassion or empathy than a plumber snaking out a drain. He may have done a dozen "insertions" that day. I was just another body.

Even after spending thirty minutes in a tiny recovery booth, and drinking a can of ginger ale, I felt stunned and woozy. I hadn't asked anyone to come to the appointment with me, because I had no idea what I was in for. Any one of my sisters would have come with me. Shoot, Baby Alice would have come down from New York if I'd asked her. My sisters and I hadn't been as close as we should be, but we showed up for each other in times of need and trouble. Baby Alice was going to give me her kidney, after all.

Now I had to get home. I had to admit I could use a hand. I thought of calling Robert at work and asking him to pick me up but decided against that idea. I'd need his help with many things soon enough.

The nurse handed me a big white plastic bag that held my clothes. I struggled to dress without moving my right side too much or bumping the contraption that now hung from a hole in my chest. I caught a glimpse of myself in the mirror and almost vomited. Instead, I swallowed hard, took a deep breath, and began walking toward the waiting room with as much dignity as I could muster. I was sure to find a cab right outside the hospital.

"Good luck, Ms. Watson," I heard the nurse call after me.

Chapter Six:
ME AND BABY ALICE

When I opened my eyes, Baby Alice was standing at my kitchen stove stir-frying vegetables in olive oil. I'd been lying on the couch for the past hour and hadn't seen the spices she added to the mix. From the aroma, I guessed Jamaican curry, celery seed, tarragon, and lots of garlic. I would have cooked those veggies the same way—except, I would have added a dash or two of pick-a-pepper—my favorite hot sauce. I'm the spicier one.

No sooner had this thought crossed my mind, than I regretted it. How insanely arrogant and condescending of me. Spicy? I didn't even have enough energy to cook for myself. That's why Alice was at my place taking care of me while I lay on the couch. Besides, where did I get off judging my sister on her level of "spiciness" anyway, whatever that meant. On February 6th, Baby Alice was going to donate one of her two precious kidneys to me. *Dine, you need to check yourself.*

Around the second week of January 2000, Baby Alice came down from her home in Highland, New York to stay with me at my apartment. I'd just started regular dialysis treatments, and while I could take care of myself, my big sister wouldn't hear of it.

"I'm not working, I have the time. Save your strength," she said.

While staying at my place, Baby Alice cooked for me every

day and prayed over me every night. Since she is a devout Seventh Day Adventist, both the food and the prayers were substantial. In addition to caring for me, Alice was traveling back and forth to the hospital to complete the tests required to be my donor. I watched my big sister cooking at my kitchen stove and wondered if I'd ever be able to ever live up to her sisterly example. Then I closed my eyes again.

"You hungry?" Alice asked, peering at me as I lay on the couch with my eyes closed. I hadn't been asleep, but I was tired. I was always tired.

Am I hungry? That was the thousand-dollar question. Since being on dialysis, I'd lost track of my taste buds. Most of the time I couldn't tell if I was hungry or not. The diet for dialysis patients is so weird. Many of the healthy foods I'd grown to love, like lots of fruits and vegetables, brown rice, beans, whole wheat bread and pasta, needed to be limited or eliminated. These foods have lots of potassium and are great for healthy people, but dangerous for someone with diminished kidney function...like me. Potassium could build up in my blood and kill me. Dr. Rudnick warned me a long time ago that dialysis did only about fifteen percent of the job the kidneys do. I remember being shocked and thinking *that's not very much*. But I suppose I had to be grateful for the dialysis machine. Until the early 1970s, when dialysis treatment became widely available in this country, a diagnosis of kidney failure was tantamount to a death sentence.

"B, you awake?" Alice asked again. "You should eat something."

I opened my eyes and looked up at my big sister. Despite how distant we'd been over the years, I loved her. We favored, she and I, with our round faces and prominent cheeks. I could see my face in hers.

"Hey, Sis," I said. "I'm awake. I'm not too hungry but I'll eat a little."

Alice looked at me sideways. She'd said something to me earlier about looking thin.

"Look, Sis," I said, giving her the side-eye right back. "The veggies smell wonderful, and I'll eat some, but I can't eat too many vegetables. Can you believe that? The nurse at the dialysis center said I'll lose body weight while on dialysis. That's what happens. The only weight I'm likely to gain is water weight, since I'm not peeing as much, so I have to watch how much I drink, too."

Alice looked at me and made a face. "TMI, TMI," she said laughing.

I laughed too. No one wanted to hear about my bathroom habits, especially not right before a meal. But we didn't laugh long. Suddenly, Baby Alice straightened her face, looked down at the floor, and shook her head.

I read her mind. "I know, Sis, I know. This is all hard to believe, isn't it? FSGS? A kidney transplant?"

My sister's face lit up again. "I'm going to trust in the Lord," she said joyfully. "Let's eat."

Baby Alice and I sat at my kitchen counter, eating silently, and looking out of the window at the blue Benjamin Franklin bridge and the night sky. Everything tasted delicious, but still, I pushed the food around my plate, like a little kid who didn't want to eat her vegetables. Had I already eaten my quota of veggies for the day? What did I have for lunch? For heaven's sake, I thought. This damn disease is going to make me afraid to eat anything.

Tuesday, Thursday, and Saturday, 9-12 noon. This was my dialysis schedule at Presbyterian Hospital's dialysis center. I was spending nine hours a week hooked up to a big, gray, whirling machine that did the job my failed kidneys could no longer do—clean my blood and keep me alive until I could have a transplant.

Baby Alice and Rob took turns driving me to and from my treatments. My sister drove me to the Center on weekdays and would instinctively take hold of my arm and help me out of the car as if I was a fragile old lady. I knew she wanted to take care of me, so I didn't dare tell her that I was perfectly capable of walking on my own. Honestly though, on some days I did feel like a fragile old lady and was grateful for my sister's attention.

On Saturdays, Robert would usually drive me to treatment. He and I would laugh, talk, and sing along to music on the car CD player until we reached Presbyterian. Then a pall would fall over us, and we'd steel ourselves for the current reality. Some mornings Robert would walk into the Center with me and help me get settled. Outsiders were not supposed to come far into the treatment room, but the staff never stopped Robert. They seemed pleased to see a young man helping his mom. On other days, however, Robert would drop me off in front of the building. I never questioned him about that choice. I assumed that on those days, he was in a hurry, or maybe the whole dialysis scene was too much for him that day—the gray walls, the hulking machines, the medical personnel scurrying about, the awful smell, and the unfortunate people that his mother would soon join, all slumped down in their big blue vinyl chairs.

I did what I could to cope. I certainly didn't want to make things worse for Baby Alice and Rob. If I was upset, I knew they would be upset. You can handle this, I told myself on every dialysis day. Things will change soon. *Trouble don't last always*, as Mommy would say. It was mid-January, and my transplant surgery was scheduled for February 6th. All I had to do was survive a few weeks of what seemed like an out-of-body experience.

Before I entered the dialysis center on my scheduled mornings, I imagined that I was surrounded by an invisible force field so strong that nothing could touch me—physically or emotionally. I followed the staff's instructions precisely: 1) weigh myself and give that number (in kilos) to my technician; 2) go to my assigned chair and put on the white gauzy gown waiting for me; 3) open my mouth and let my technician take my temperature; 4) stick out my arm and let my technician apply the blood pressure cup and take my blood pressure and finally, the big one, 5) allow the technician to clean my chest with a cold, iodine-like solution, and hook the tubes coming out of my chest to the tubes connected to the dialysis machine. Then I'd settle back into my blue chair and think, "Let the blood cleansing begin."

I never counted them, but I believe there were at least fifty dialysis machines in that room, each positioned next to a blue chair. During my three-hour shift, almost all the chairs were filled—with other Black people. The machines and chairs were arranged in two semi-circles on either side of a large medical station where the clinic managers sat. My chair was in the middle of the first row on the far side of the room. If I chose to, I could see everyone who came through the Center door and everything that happened at the medical station. However, instead of watching the room, I chose to watch the clock on the front wall and paid little attention to what was going on around me. I was polite, but most days, all I could manage was a nod in the direction of anyone I encountered. This included the people who sat on either side of me during my shift, and the technicians whose job it was to hook me up to the machine. As far as I was concerned, I was just passing through. I don't belong here, I thought. I don't need to get to know anyone. Besides watching the clock, I did my time with a good book or, if I was lucky, on the wings of a good dream.

During the weeks Baby Alice spent at my place, we ate many meals together at my kitchen counter, most of them made by her hands. Sometimes the only sound in my apartment was me and my sister chewing and murmuring in appreciation of the good food. Often, I'd sneak a look at my sister and wonder: when was the last time Alice and I spent this much time together? On some evenings, I remembered the two of us as much younger—sitting next to each other at the family dining room table; listening to music and dancing the cha-cha in the kitchen when we were supposed to be doing the dishes; walking to the bookmobile to check out library books and singing together in the Tindley Temple youth choir. But over the decades our lives had gone in such different directions. Now here we were, sisters side by side again. But sometimes the feeling between us was both intimate and strange. What were we supposed to talk about?

One night, Baby Alice must have felt the strangeness too. I turned to find her watching me intently.

"Why don't you put on some music?" she said abruptly. "Put on Morgana King."

"Damn!" I cursed under my breath. No matter how old I was I still did not curse in front of my older sister. Why did she have to ask for one of the jazz singers whose music I didn't have? I liked Morgana King and was happy to hear her on the radio now and then, but she wasn't a favorite. Her voice was a bit operatic for me. Now I regretted not having at least one of her discs. According to my reputation in the family, I was the one who was into jazz, the one with the vast music collection; the "spicy" one. Now I couldn't fill a simple music request.

"I'm sorry, Alice," I said frowning. "I don't have Morgana King. I have Nancy, Sarah, Betty, Billie, Ella, Abbey, and many others. Remember when we used to listen to Gloria Lynne—*The Folks Who Live on the Hill*? I know you like Gloria Lynne."

Baby Alice looked at me as if I'd committed a mortal sin. "You don't have Morgana King? I thought you had everything," she responded. I think she was joking, but I thought I also heard a bit of facetiousness in her voice—*What kind of jazz diva doesn't have Morgana King in her collection?*

"Look, Sis," I said with a shrug. "Let me play something for you. I guarantee you'll enjoy it."

Without waiting for her response, I headed over to the CD player and filled the changer with Nancy Wilson and Sarah Vaughan. What's not to like? I decided to leave the more eclectic voices of Abbey Lincoln and Betty Carter, my current favorites, out of the mix for the time being. The silence in my apartment melted away as Nancy and Sarah sassed the room. In no time my big sister and I were talking, laughing, and remembering our youth.

"Remember how we used to listen to the radio in the kitchen all the time?" I asked. "Remember those DJs—Georgie Woods—The Man with the Goods, Jocko, and Jimmy Bishop?"

"Who could forget that kitchen," Alice responded, laughing. "The floor was practically made of dirt. No matter how many times I swept it I couldn't get the thing clean."

"Isn't that the truth," I laughed, since I also had tried to clean that kitchen floor. But I wanted to keep the conversation on music, something I knew Alice and I had both loved as girls.

"Remember the great music the jocks used to play—The Shirelles, The Marvelettes, the Chantelles, Smokey Robinson and the Miracles? We used to love that stuff."

The truth is my big sister Baby Alice had introduced me to those old soul groups. She'd been a big part of my learning to love that music.

"Do you still listen to music?" I asked her, wondering if her religious practice meant no music.

"Sometimes," Baby Alice said. "I mostly sing in my church choir."

I didn't respond to my sister, since I didn't know what to say. I missed the Baby Alice who loved soul music and dancing as much as I did. Again, silence filled the apartment. As if on cue, Baby Alice looked around my apartment at my well-chosen furniture, art, and carefully curated objects and said,

"B, you've done all right for yourself. You've come a long way from those days on Montrose Street. I'm proud of you."

"Thank you, Sis," I said, grateful to have her admiration. Still, I wondered if we'd ever be as close as we once were. I didn't know, so I let Sarah's voice fill the room.

∽

"How are you, Ms. Watson?"

I'd been half asleep in my dialysis chair when Dr. Rudnick's voice startled me. I didn't know he'd be making weekly rounds in the Center and certainly hadn't expected to see him that morning. As I opened my eyes and saw him standing over me, I began to recall how, in my opinion, he hadn't adequately prepared me for the whole dialysis process—from having my catheter installed to how tired I would feel after a treatment.

"Hi, Ms. Watson," Dr. Rudnick repeated. "How are you adjusting to dialysis? Your labs look pretty good."

"I'm holding up, Dr. Rudnick," I said. I was trying to hold my anger in and could feel my heart starting to race.

Finally, I blurted, "Why didn't you tell me that I was going to have a catheter inserted when you sent me to Intervention Radiology? I had no idea. If I'd known, I would have asked someone to come with me."

Rudnick looked puzzled, surprised, and annoyed all at once. He shifted his wiry frame from one foot to the other and appeared uncomfortable for a moment.

"Ms. Watson, I told you that you would need dialysis. I didn't think it wise to wait. You can get extremely sick if your creatinine level gets too high. I apologize if there was some misunderstanding."

As I listened to Rudnick, I realized that it was futile to continue this discussion. He didn't seem to have any idea why I was upset. Besides, I was sitting in a dialysis chair with needles in my chest that were attached to a machine. Maybe this wasn't the best time to get upset. I'd been on dialysis for over a week and was doing okay. I decided to try and push the horrible experience with Intervention Radiology to the back of my mind.

Dr. Rudnick was still looking down at me. I supposed he was waiting for me to respond to his apology.

"I'm hanging in there, Dr. Rudnick. I only have a few weeks to go before my transplant."

"Yes, yes," Rudnick said, sounding as excited as I'd ever heard him. "I've been in touch with Dr. Bloom, over at Penn Transplant, and he says everything's on track for early February. How's your sister?"

"We're both good," I responded. My heart was still pounding so I took a few deep breaths. I wanted my pulse and blood pressure to be normal when he took my vitals.

"She's finished her testing here in Philadelphia and everything looks good. We're ready to go."

"Good, good. Let me listen to your heart, please," he said, pulling a stethoscope from his pocket.

Satisfied with what he heard, Rudnick patted me on the arm. "I'll see you next week."

As if Dr. Rudnick's visit wasn't enough to wreck my calm that morning, I had another issue on my mind. I was only a few weeks away from my transplant surgery and hadn't told my mother that I had kidney disease, let alone that both Baby Alice and I were about to undergo major surgery. I didn't want to tell her anything at all. My big sister disagreed.

"How in the world are we going to keep something like this from Mommy?" she asked me with her hands on her hips and her head whipping from side to side in true South Philly girl style.

I shrugged my shoulders, but I knew the answer to Alice's question. Just don't tell her. My sister didn't know how many secrets I'd kept from Mommy and the rest of the family over the years, like the hysterectomy I had in 1995. I learned my lesson many years ago when I was nineteen years old and had to tell Mommy I was pregnant. Don't bring Mommy no bad news.

"We won't be in the hospital that long and then we just need a couple of months to recuperate. She doesn't have to find out. We don't see her that often anyway. You know how Mommy can be when she gets upset. She lost Daddy not too long ago."

"We have to tell her," Alice insisted. "I talked to Cousin Jeanie yesterday and she agrees with me. With two of her children going under the knife, Mommy deserves to know. Look, we'll tell her the problem, but we can also tell her the solution. You need a transplant, but you have a donor. Me. C'mon, B, that's the best thing to do."

I let out a loud sigh and stared at my sister. Why did she

have to bring Jeanie into this? Jeanie is our older cousin. She was raised by Grandma Daisy and grew up next door to us. She was practically an older sister. Her opinion carried a lot of weight. I was outnumbered.

"Okay, okay," I relented. "Let's go right now, then."

I watched Alice carefully. Would she take me up on my offer? Before I could take my eyes off her, she headed quickly toward the hallway closet for her coat.

"Okay, let's go," she said, handing me my coat too as if she was worried that I might change my mind. She was right to worry.

Mommy was in the kitchen when we came in the door.

"Hi, sweethearts," she said, joyfully coming out of the kitchen and wiping her hands on her apron. Mommy would tell you in a minute that she wasn't a great cook, but I could smell the pungent scent of cabbage and white potatoes cooking—one of Mommy's favorite dishes. My heart leaped for a moment. I was happy to see Mommy downstairs and cooking. She'd spent so much time in bed since Daddy died. Then I remembered why we were at the house and my heart fell again.

"Hi, Mommy," Alice and I said almost simultaneously, both of us putting our arms around her. The group hug felt good.

"Ali, I didn't know you were here. When did you come down?"

I glanced at my sister and waited to hear what she was going to say.

"I've been down for a few days visiting B," she said, telling a version of the truth.

"Is Lin here?" I asked quickly, to change the subject. My sister Linda and her husband were moving into my parents' house. Mommy couldn't stay in the house by herself after Daddy died and they'd agreed to rent out their house in South Philly and move in with Ma.

"Yes, she's upstairs, God bless her," Mommy said shaking her head. She was so thankful to Linda. We all were. Her sacrifice solved one big problem for the family. Now here I was with another one.

"Lin, come down, your sisters are here," she called up the back staircase.

In a few seconds, Linda came running down the stairs. As children, we learned to come running when Mommy or Daddy called. During another group hug, I realized that we should have let Linda in on what was about to happen. Too late now.

"Why don't we all go sit at the dining room table? I have something to tell you," I said.

Mommy turned her head sharply to look at me. Linda gave me a knowing look. Even if we hadn't given her a heads up today, she knew this day would come.

"What's the matter, B?" Mommy asked. I could hear the alarm rising in her voice.

"I'm so sorry, Mommy. I'm so sorry, Mommy," I whispered under my breath.

"Why don't we sit down," I said again, taking my mother's arm and guiding her toward the dining room. Mom sat at the head of the table while Linda, Alice, and I sat on either side. No one took the seat at the other end where Daddy would have undoubtedly been.

"Mom, I need a kidney transplant," I said. No sense in making small talk.

"What?" she said, looking genuinely puzzled. I couldn't tell if she hadn't heard me, or if she didn't understand what I said.

I repeated myself more slowly and then immediately

launched into the explanation of FSGS and everything I'd been through up to this point. I knew the speech by heart by now. I'd said the words a thousand times. But this was Mommy and I tried to speak with care. I was telling her that one of the children she'd brought into the world had a life-threatening illness. I certainly would not want to hear anything like that from Robert.

When I finished my story, my mother stared at me for a moment and asked a question I hadn't expected. "You said you need a kidney transplant. Don't we have two kidneys? I know some people who were born with one. If one of yours is bad, why can't you use the other one?"

Mommy looked around the table at each of us. Her wide eyes challenged us to answer her question. Linda and Alice both looked at me as if to say—"Well, answer her."

I sat silently at first, not sure I knew the answer to her question. Then I told her what I thought was the truth.

"My kidney system has failed, Ma. I have end-stage renal disease. Both kidneys are bad."

I'd lived with the reality of my kidney failure now for several weeks, but the words end-stage renal disease still sounded horrible. I hated to use those words, but the term unambiguously communicated the seriousness of my situation. Mommy got the message. She put her head down on the dining room table and wept as hard as she had when Daddy died. None of us tried to quiet her.

∼

BABY ALICE and I arrived at the University of Pennsylvania hospital on Sunday, February 5, 2000, early in the evening. We came with a caravan, including Mommy, my sister Linda, Rob, and Kathleen—one of the friends from Minneapolis who I'd told about my illness when I was first diagnosed in 1986. Kathleen and I had remained friends over the miles and years, and she'd put her life on hold to be with me during the surgery.

The medical staff at Penn welcomed us like conquering heroes. By 2000, kidney transplants had been performed for over forty years, but the doctors and nurses treated my sister and me as if we were part of a new and exciting medical discovery. The nurses fussed over us as we settled into our rooms, and the transplant team patiently talked with my family in the hallway about FSGS disease and walked them through the surgery. I overheard one of the surgeons explain tell my mother,

"There's a lot we don't understand about FSGS. It's a brutal disease and can recur in a transplanted kidney. One thing we do know is that FSGS is much more common in African Americans than in White people."

The doctor paused for a minute as if to let my mother absorb that information. *It can recur in a transplanted kidney.* Then he added, "Don't worry, Mrs. Hayes, a kidney transplant is the best way to extend your daughter's life. She's healthy and her sister is a perfect match. We're going to take good care of both your daughters."

I couldn't see my mother's face, but so far, she'd held up well. I'd asked Rob to keep a special eye on her just in case.

My sister and I were given single rooms, which was standard procedure for transplant patients, because of the risk of infection. I thought Baby Alice would be in a room close to me, but for some unexplainable reason, she was down at the other end of the hallway. My family did their best to divide their time evenly between us. Kathleen and I made nervous small talk in my room. Everyone seemed tired and tense as if the seriousness of the surgery was suddenly sinking in. By around 8 p.m. when everyone was gone and I was alone in my hospital room, I realized how exhausted, tense, and scared I was. An icy shiver ran down my spine as I thought, tomorrow morning a surgeon is going to cut my sister's body open and take out her kidney. Another surgeon will cut my body open and put my sister's kidney inside me. Then we'd all hope and pray that everything would be okay.

I lay down in the hospital bed and pulled the thin sheet and blanket up over me. Immediately I realized that I was freezing. I needed another blanket, or maybe two, and pulled the cord for the nurse.

"Yes, Ms. Watson, can I help you?"

"Can I please have another blanket?" I asked through chattering teeth.

The nurse came over to the bed to take a closer look at me. She scrunched her face with concern, then put the back of her hand on my forehead.

"Ms. Watson, I think you have a fever," she said, sounding shocked. "When did all this happen?" She reached for a thermometer. I wanted to tell the nurse that I had no idea what was happening. I'd felt fine all day. I just needed a blanket. The nurse took the thermometer from my mouth and shook her head. "My goodness, Ms. Watson. You have a fever of 101. I'm calling Dr. Bloom."

"Could you please bring me a blanket?" I asked weakly as she hurried out of the room.

I'd hardly gotten the words out of my mouth when my stomach began to lurch. I stumbled toward the bathroom, just making it to the toilet before I vomited all over the place.

What the hell is going on? I'd heard about hospitals making you sick, but never thought it would happen to me the night before my transplant. I was fine a few hours ago. Now I felt horrible. I walked gingerly back to the bed and crawled in. If I could rest, I'd be okay.

"Ms. Watson, it's Dr. Bloom."

A hand pressed lightly on my arm. When I opened my eyes, all I could see was a blur of White faces and white coats. A few seconds passed before I remembered where I was and what was happening. I smelled like vomit.

Two young men stood beside Dr. Bloom, both looking unsure about whether they should look directly at me. Since Penn is a teaching hospital, I assumed they were med students or interns. I hated being a living specimen on display, especially since I was sure I had vomit stuck to my face.

"Ms. Watson, I hear you're not feeling well. What's going on?" Bloom folded his arms across his chest and looked down at me.

"I have no idea what's wrong. I was fine when I came in this afternoon, then suddenly a few minutes ago I started to feel ill."

Dr. Bloom frowned, sat down on the side of the bed, and leaned in close. He took a pin light out of his pocket.

"Open your eyes wide, Ms. Watson," he said, shining light in my right eye and then my left.

Bloom turned to one of the younger doctors, "Please ask one of the nurses to come in and help Ms. Watson get cleaned up."

Immediately, one of the young men scurried out of the room. I looked up at Dr. Bloom expectantly. He let out a long sigh and patted my arm again.

"I think, unfortunately, you've contracted a bug, Ms. Watson. Either something you came in here with or something you caught since you've been here. I'll ask the nurse to take your temperature again, but you feel warm. I'm sure you still have a fever. Do you have an infection that you know of? Are there any open sores on your body?"

I managed to shake my pounding head "no."

"I'm sorry, Ms. Watson," Dr. Bloom said. "This is probably not serious. I can see you feel lousy and I'm going to get out of here so the nurse can clean you up and you can sleep. But here's the deal. We'll have to keep an eye on you. Tonight, we need to start your immunosuppressants so your body will accept your sister's kidney tomorrow. But if you still have a fever in a few hours, we'll have to postpone the surgery. We can't do the transplant if you're sick."

I watched Dr. Bloom's lips move but didn't want to accept the words coming out of his mouth. No transplant? After all this? I wanted more of an explanation from him, but I felt too sick to keep talking.

In addition to cleaning me up, the nurse gave me some medicine to help settle my stomach and bring my fever down. I began to give myself a pep talk: *Listen, Dine. Try to get some sleep. Sleep will help. You'll feel much better in the morning, and they'll go through with the surgery. Get some rest, Get some rest.* I repeated the words like a mantra or lullaby.

Between nurses whizzing in and out taking my temperature and blood pressure, the beeping and bumping of the nighttime hospital right outside my door, and my pounding head, I couldn't sleep or even rest much. More than anything, I worried about what the morning might or might not bring. What if they send me home without the surgery? I'll have to go back to dialysis. And what about Baby Alice? She's been here in Philly for over a month and now the surgery might be canceled. I wonder if they've told her anything. *Please, please, please*, I begged whoever might be listening.

I must have drifted off to sleep at some point because I awakened to daylight streaming into the hospital room window and to an unfamiliar voice.

"Good morning, Ms. Watson, I'm Dr. Anu, one of the transplant surgeons. How are you feeling this morning?"

I looked at the clock on the wall across from my bed. A little before 7:00. I then turned to look at Dr. Anu who I hadn't met before. He looked East-Indian with skin the color of a chestnut, and silvery gray hair that fell against the shoulders of his white lab coat. He too was trailed by medical students, who looked positively pallid in his presence. This time there were three of them—all White, but one was a woman.

"Good morning. I feel better than I did yesterday," I said, trying to sound cheerful and alert.

"The nurses were in and out all night," I continued. Did they give me the anti-rejection medicine already?"

I don't think Dr. Anu will ever know how disappointed I was by his response.

"I'm sorry Ms. Watson," Dr. Anu said kindly, sounding honestly sorry, but still firm and direct. "We won't be able to go through with the transplant surgery today. Earlier this morning when we checked your temperature, you still had a fever. A fever can cause all kinds of complications with surgery, especially if we don't know exactly what's causing it. We just can't take that risk. We've canceled the transplant for today and will try to get you and your sister back on schedule as soon as possible. You'll be going home today."

I stared at the kind doctor giving me this unkind news. Tears welled up in my eyes. My head started to pound again and for the first time since I woke up, I realized that I still felt hot. I still had a fever.

At first, I tried as hard as I could to keep from crying but was surprised that I couldn't keep the tears from rolling down my face. One part of me was horrified that I had lost all control in front of these doctors. Another part of me wanted to go crazy and start screaming. The whole situation felt like a nightmare—me having FSGS in the first place, Baby Alice waiting down the hall to have her body cut open, me getting sick in the hospital, this long-awaited surgery now being canceled on the morning of. I didn't scream, but I couldn't stop crying.

"Please calm down, Ms. Watson," Dr. Anu said gently as he handed me a tissue from the bedside table. He turned to one of the young doctors and said, "Please bring Ms. Watson a glass of water."

With a few sips of water, my mind began to clear. After a few more sips I could feel my body start to relax and the scream in my chest ease. The tears, however, kept falling, although I wiped them away as quickly as I could.

Dr. Anu watched patiently as I tried to pull myself together. The three young doctors seemed to stare at me with curiosity. I wondered if they'd ever seen a Black woman cry.

"We'll do everything we can to get you back into surgery as soon as possible, Ms. Watson," said Dr. Anu sincerely.

I believed the doctor, but the idea of going home without my new kidney still seemed unbearable.

"Dr. Anu," I asked, "is it possible for me to stay in the hospital for a few days until I'm well enough to have the surgery? I should be over this bug in a few days at the most."

I already knew the answer to my question. My insurance would never pay for me to stay in the hospital unnecessarily. The irony of begging for a surgery I'd tried so hard to avoid seemed almost pitiful. I felt pitiful anyway, so what difference did it make?

"Ms. Watson, that's not possible," the doctor said. "You and your sister should go home and get some rest. You'll probably feel better at home anyway. Of course, go see your primary if you're not feeling better in a few days. Okay?"

I wasn't okay, but I was done crying.

"Has someone spoken with my sister?"

One of the student doctors answered.

"I think someone is talking with her now." The thought of Baby Alice's disappointment made me feel even worse.

"Get some rest, Ms. Watson," Anu said flashing a smile. "Keep your spirits up. Stick with your dialysis schedule and the hospital will be in touch. We'll see each other again soon."

The surgeon turned and left the room. The three students followed a respectable distance behind him.

My friend Kathleen, who'd left a toddler and husband at home, flew back to Minneapolis on the day I left the hospital. Baby Alice decided to go back home to Highland and wait until the hospital gave us a new date. I didn't blame her. She'd been away from her family for a long time. My sister had been a tremendous help to me, and her visit had given us needed time together. But now that I was somewhat used to the dialysis treatments, I could cook for myself and even get to and from the Center by myself, even if I had to take a cab every day. Cabs were expensive, but I didn't care. The time to spend money is when you need to take care of yourself. If not now, when? Besides, I knew that Rob would help as much as he could.

The truth is, if I had to be sent home, I wanted to be alone in my apartment. Being alone was familiar, almost comforting. I needed time to nurse my disappointment about the canceled surgery and mentally prepare for the transplant all over again. I wanted to stare out my living room window at my big blue bridge and dream about a time when this transplant business would be behind me.

I'd gone to the hospital on Sunday afternoon, February 5, expecting to have a kidney transplant the next morning. By Tuesday morning, February 8, I was back at the dialysis center waiting for someone to hook me up to a machine. The bug that attacked me in the hospital and postponed my transplant surgery was almost gone, except for the fatigue I still felt. The fatigue was nothing new though. I'd been tired for a long time.

I felt sheepish walking back into the dialysis center. Word had gotten around that I was having a transplant. When I left the Center after what was supposed to be my last treatment, a few patients even wished me luck. Now here I was back in my blue chair. However, no one seemed to notice when I walked in and took my seat. I supposed these folks had their own problems and didn't have time for mine.

I caught a glimpse of Dr. Rudnick making rounds. Just my luck. I wasn't ready for Rudnick. I closed my eyes and pretended to be asleep, but that made no difference.

"Good morning, Ms. Watson. I didn't expect to see you here."

I opened my eyes to Dr. Rudnick standing beside my chair.

"I thought you'd be in the hospital getting transplanted," he said. "What happened?"

Don't you doctors talk to each other, I wondered. I wasn't interested in telling the story of "the transplant that didn't happen." All I wanted was to do my three hours on the machine and get out of this place. However, Dr. Rudnick was standing in my personal space waiting for me to answer his question.

"Well, Dr. Rudnick," I began slowly, "my surgery was supposed to be yesterday, but I got sick while I was in the hospital.

TRANSPLANT: A MEMOIR

I was vomiting and had a fever. The transplant surgery had to be canceled."

Rudnick made a face I couldn't quite decipher and began to pull his stethoscope out of his pocket.

"How are you feeling now?" he asked.

"Much better, thank you," I responded, as I carefully shifted my body toward the front of the chair. Dr. Rudnick needed to reach me with the stethoscope. On the other hand, I had to make sure that my movement didn't knock the dialysis tubes out of my chest. Blood would fly everywhere. I'd seen it happen.

"The doctors think it was a bug. I guess I had one of those 24-hour bugs since I was sick for about 24 hours—long enough so my surgery was canceled." I sighed with disgust.

Dr. Rudnick looked at me and chuckled. "Ms. Watson, you must be snake bitten."

Snake bitten. What the hell is "snake bitten?" I had no idea what Rudnick was talking about, but I knew I didn't like him laughing about my surgery being postponed. I closed my eyes and sat as still as I could so he could listen to my heart and lungs. That was all that mattered.

When I got home, I looked up "snake bitten" on the internet: *Someone who has been characterized by bad luck or a series of misfortunes.* Rudnick's comment annoyed me, but he wasn't wrong.

The transplant was rescheduled for March 3, about a month after the first surgery was canceled. I spent the month lying low, sleeping, reading, doing yoga, and going to my dialysis treatments. I also took a meditation class at a neighborhood spa. When I asked the class leader if meditating would help me get through the transplant surgery and heal well, he replied, "We can be hopeful." I was.

Baby Alice stayed at my apartment the night before the surgery. In the morning we dressed without speaking much. What else was there to say? Linda drove downtown and took us to the hospital. Mommy didn't come with us. I imagined her at home on her knees asking her God to take care of her two daughters.

The staff didn't fuss over us much this time. Everyone, including Alice and me seemed determined to get the job done. Thoughts about the surgery being postponed a second time were never far from my mind. Around midnight, when the nurse came in to administer the immunosuppressant drugs, I began to feel confident that that transplant would take place the next day. I lay awake in the dark feeling frightened and vulnerable. My immune system had been suppressed so my body could accept an organ that didn't belong inside me. Eventually, I fell asleep.

The next morning, Baby Alice and I lay side by side on gurneys outside separate operating rooms. We held hands and laughed at how silly we looked in our surgical hats. I felt so close to her. She was my big sister. We'd only been waiting a few minutes when an orderly walked up and announced, "Alice Cook, you're first." My stomach jolted. The surgeon had explained that Alice would be operated on first, so her kidney would be waiting for me. Still, I wasn't quite ready to see my sister wheeled away.

I squeezed Alice's hand and made a "scary" face like the ones we used to make when we were kids. Only this time we weren't playing. Alice squeezed my hand back and mouthed her trusted mantra—"everything's going to be okay."

Chapter Seven:
GET YOURSELF TOGETHER

After the transplant surgery, Baby Alice and I went our separate ways to recover. She went to my parents' home. I went to my apartment. My mother was not happy about my decision.

"But B," Mommy moaned into the telephone beside my hospital bed. "You shouldn't be in that apartment alone. You've had major surgery. How are you going to take care of yourself?"

I understood where Mommy was coming from. I knew she was looking forward to nursing her two girls back to health. I also sensed that she needed someone else to focus on besides Daddy, who'd been dead for almost a year. A part of me wanted to go to Mommy's house. Baby Alice and I might have fun. I fantasized briefly about Alice and me lying in bed on the second floor, laughing, gossiping, and watching TV like girls, waiting for Mommy to bring us chicken soup, ice cream, or whatever we wanted. However, my fantasy was a true fantasy. There were no scenes like this in my real childhood. Even if there were, my sister and I weren't children anymore.

"I'm fine, Mommy," I said, trying my best to sound "fine" rather than still exhausted from the surgery. "The elevator in my building will take me up to my apartment. Everything in my place is on one floor, and I feel strong enough to prepare my own food. If I don't want to cook, I'll have food delivered or ask Robert to make something for me. You know Rob will look after me, Mommy."

I didn't tell her that my man friend, Ed, who'd kept me company throughout the year before the surgery and still came by from time to time, was all too happy to look in on me.

Mommy didn't say anything. I recognized her deafening silence. She was hurt and probably frustrated with me. *I'm the child who always disappoints her,* I thought.

Still, I knew what was good for me. I needed time to absorb the surgery and figure out how to put my life back together. To recover, I needed to be in my own home, surrounded by my own books and artwork, listening to my own music, eating my own food, and staring at the big blue bridge outside my living room window. In the thirty-plus years since I'd left home as a scared, pregnant girl, I'd deliberately built my own life— separate from my family. I was certain that getting back to my life was what would help me heal.

I loved the time my sister Baby Alice and I had spent together before the transplant. We'd needed that time. Still, I didn't want another week of "working" on a relationship with my sister when I was supposed to be recovering. Years later, when talking about the surgery, I asked Alice if she thought I should have come home to Mommy's to recover with her. She answered emphatically, "No. That would have been too much for Mommy. She couldn't take care of both of us."

My sister's response made me glad I followed my own mind.

Telling my mother that I was fine though, was an exaggeration. The incision on the right side of my stomach, where the surgeon tucked my new kidney, was still painful, especially when I coughed, laughed, or moved suddenly. However, I had plenty of Percocet and Oxycodone to keep me from feeling too much pain. Hell, I soon found out that the real pain was extreme constipation caused by these medications. After a few days, I traded the opioids for Extra Strength Tylenol which meant increased pain from the incision. However, the trade-off was worth it. I regained the ability to "handle my business," and standing up straight became at least bearable.

I decided to take advantage of all the sick and disability leave I had and told my office I'd be out for at least six months. Dr. Rudnick thought that it was excessive, to say the least.

"Six months," he scoffed in disbelief. "Most kidney transplant patients are back to work in six weeks. I see this all the time."

I didn't let Rudnick's reaction intimidate me. He might have treated a lot of patients but hadn't gone through a kidney transplant. He had no idea what I was dealing with.

I wasn't a fool, though. I understood that six months was a long time to be away from a job. I didn't know if I'd have a position to go back to or even if I'd want to return. I needed to heal physically, emotionally, and mentally. The last year had been hell. I'd take my chances.

Fortunately, one of the other doctors on my transplant team was willing to sign the disability papers allowing me to take six months off from work. My boss wasn't crazy about my absence for that long either, but he accepted it. I had a doctor's note.

I spent my days waking in the morning whenever my body was ready, taking naps whenever I felt sleepy, and going to bed at night when I decided my day was done. I took long, luxurious showers, a pleasure I'd given up while on dialysis. If the dialysis catheter hanging out of my chest had gotten wet, I'd have risked a blood infection. When I was on dialysis, I'd reduced my daily bathing routine to washing up at the bathroom sink. Having to stand naked and shivering at the sink reminded me of my childhood. My sisters and I would line up at the bathtub and wash up over tin basins. No one in our neighborhood of tiny Philly row houses had a shower. Most houses, including ours, didn't even have a sink in the bathroom—just a toilet and tub. What a joy to stand under the shower head again and feel hot water flow all over my body.

I also took time to familiarize myself with the voluminous amount of medicine I now had to take to keep my new kidney healthy. The immunosuppressant medications—Tacrolimus and Cellcept—suppressed my immune system, diminishing the chance that my body would reject my new kidney.

According to Dr. Rudnick, "As far as your body is concerned, your new kidney is a foreign object. Without these medications, your immune system will do its job and try to get rid of it."

Prednisone, a steroid, reduced the inflammation in my body that could also cause the rejection of my kidney. While I'd been taking blood pressure medication before my transplant, I now needed a larger dose since the immunosuppressants could cause my blood pressure to run higher. Add to these medications a statin to help control my cholesterol and an antibiotic to help ward off infections I was now susceptible to because of a suppressed immune system, and I was taking thirteen pills a day. Before I left the hospital, the nurse gave me all my medicines in a large plastic case that could hold a week's worth of pills.

"I know this looks like a lot of pills," she laughed, "but believe me, I have AIDS patients who take many more pills than this."

I just stared at her. I didn't find AIDS or kidney disease very funny.

TRANSPLANT: A MEMOIR

Initially, I thought I had everything under control. Every Sunday evening, while sitting at my kitchen counter watching the news or *60 Minutes*, I took out my plastic case. Then I'd sort the next seven days' worth of medication into the little boxes marked with the time of day I was to take each dose. The container helped, and being a disciplined person, I quickly developed a regimen of taking my medicine as prescribed. I was proud of myself and felt that my old confidence was returning.

However, after a few weeks of this regimen, when I began to feel the side effects of these powerful pharmaceuticals, nothing felt under my control. Almost every day, the medicines elicited a range of reactions from my body—trembling, nausea, diarrhea, fatigue, anxiety, and mood swings.

"Ms. Watson," the doctors explained, "you're feeling the effects of the immunosuppressants and the steroid. This is not unusual. We're giving you the lowest dose of each that we can—any lower and you'll risk rejection. Your body will get used to the medicines. Take Nexium for your stomach and Imodium for diarrhea. Things should settle down."

One side effect of the Prednisone was the fat deposits the medicines left on my cheeks, neck, and stomach—all the places a girl wants fat, right? I'd inherited chubby cheeks from my mom's side of the family and never liked the rounded look they gave my face. What woman didn't want chiseled cheekbones? But I thought the Prednisone made me look like a chipmunk. Even kidney doctors use the "medical" term, "chipmunk cheeks," or "moon face" to describe the effect Prednisone has on the face.

"Everyone hates Prednisone," the doctors told me. They were right. I once overheard another transplant patient refer to the drug as "the devil's friend." The doctor's advice to me was watch your diet and reduce your salt intake. Nothing helped.

Another unkind cut was that my eyes, the "windows to my soul," still had a reddish tinge. I'd suffered from unhealthy-looking, red eyes before the transplant but thought they were part of the overall effect FSGS was having on my body. I'd hoped mightily that my new kidney would cleanse these impurities from my blood and restore the whites of my eyes to their whiteness. Unfortunately, my eyes still reflected a shadowy redness that no amount of sleep or eye drops diminished. Since my transplant doctors couldn't explain the persistent redness, I decided that all the new medicines were the culprit. I hated the impact these medicines were having on my face and started leaving the bathroom cabinet door open, so I wouldn't have to see my reflection in the mirror.

Nevertheless, it seemed that as far as the transplant team was concerned, I was a walking miracle. The medicines that kept my transplant working were among the greatest advances in medical history. When I went to the transplant clinic for checkups, nurses called out to me in cheery voices,

"Hi, Ms. Watson, looking good! How's your sister?"

Doctors gathered to see my lab work and commented to each other proudly, "Look at those numbers."

Everyone made sympathetic noises in response to my concerns but did little to help me feel better.

"You're on the right doses of medication. You look good, and your creatinine level is great." Then they'd give that dire warning, "If we reduce your medicines, you could have a rejection episode."

I didn't disagree with my medical team. I was grateful for everything. Having a new kidney *was* a miracle. Having a sister like Baby Alice *was* a miracle. Having a life without dialysis *was* a miracle. I was truly grateful!

Still, the exchanges with my doctors left me feeling helpless and unheard. Of course, I didn't want to lose my new kidney—not after everything Baby Alice and I had been through. My sister had her body cut open for me, for goodness' sake. But that didn't mean I wanted to walk around looking like a fat-faced, nervous wreck.

I got the impression that the doctors thought I was a drama queen. Was I a little vain? Maybe, but what's wrong with me being concerned about my appearance? I wanted someone on the transplant team who would listen and understand my feelings. A nutritionist, a social worker, a therapist, someone. There didn't seem to be anyone.

What's more, my appearance wasn't my only worry. With every post-operative visit, I learned more about the seriousness of living with a transplanted organ inside my body:

"Ms. Watson, make sure you take your medicines exactly as prescribed, or you could have a rejection episode."

"Ms. Watson, these medications are designed to keep your transplant working but they also lower your immunity to other diseases like diabetes and cancer. Make sure you keep up with pap smears, dental checkups, and other screenings."

"Ms. Watson, the FSGS can recur in your new kidney at any time, and there is little we can do besides another transplant if the disease comes back."

Recurrence! Rejection! Cancer! In addition to concern about my appearance, and the side effects I was experiencing from the medications, those words began to invade my every thought. I felt woefully unprepared for life after my transplant. Why didn't I know what to expect after this surgery? Did I miss the talk from my doctors about the downsides of a kidney transplant? Was I so wrapped up in wanting to be free of dialysis and back in control of my life that I didn't hear the cautions? What's more, where was the iron will I'd always depended on? Had I come undone?

These questions and concerns swirled in my head like a dust storm. I wasn't questioning the wisdom of the surgery. I couldn't survive a life of dialysis. Thank goodness for Baby Alice. But I was now living in a brand-new reality.

For weeks, I lay on the sofa in my living room: popping pills, reading, listening to music, staring out of the window, and watching T.V., leaving home primarily to keep doctors' appointments. By sometime in May, I could feel myself beginning to mend physically. My incision had healed without complications and I was handling any physical discomfort with over-the-counter medication. My stomach had stopped lurching, the diarrhea lessened, and my blood pressure had settled into the normal range.

But emotionally, I was still reeling. I hated my puffy face. My hands shook. Any little upset could reduce me to tears, and I never knew if I was going to wake up mad, sad, or glad. The transplant doctors assured me that my feelings were a reaction to the medications. Repeatedly they told me, "You're doing great," "You'll get used to the meds," and "You'll be fine."

I didn't feel great or fine and didn't know if I ever would again. On some days I'd lay on my sofa paralyzed with feelings of fear and embarrassment that my body had failed me so spectacularly. I'd ask myself, "Do you know anyone else your age who's been on dialysis or had a kidney transplant?" The answer was always no.

Few people besides Robert and my friend Ed came by to visit—Robert to bring food and to try and cheer me up; Ed to keep me company for a while. I didn't want visitors, anyway. I didn't feel ready for the world. Many of the people in my life didn't even know I'd been ill or had a transplant. I'd tell who I wanted to tell later when the whole freaking episode was over.

I thought a lot about my sister Alice as I lay on the couch. She and I had spoken only a few times since we left the hospital. I knew I should call her. I hoped she wasn't in any pain. I knew my sister wouldn't suffer the same medicinal side effects that I did, but she'd been through a huge trauma too. And now she was down to one kidney. All because of me. I told myself that I didn't feel like talking and she probably didn't either. Didn't we both need our rest?

Spring dwindled into summer, and I moved from lying on the sofa all day to sitting up, to eventually leaving my apartment for walks or to sit in my building's courtyard. As I regained my strength, I sometimes walked to the Reading Terminal for groceries. Occasionally, I answered calls from people other than Rob, Ed, or my mom and even began meeting close friends occasionally for coffee or lunch. But when I was outside of my apartment, I felt vulnerable and ill at ease. Could people smell the illness on me? See the Prednisone in my chipmunk cheeks?

The only time I felt truly comfortable was in my living room listening to my music. Music has always been my saving grace, my sanctuary. Over the years, I'd amassed over a thousand CDs —mostly jazz, but including almost every genre. I started many of my "sofa days" asking: What do you want to listen to, girlie? What will make you feel better? Do you need a voice? A horn? A lovely piano melody? Something wild? Something peaceful? An oldie but goodie?

My CD collection was arranged alphabetically by artist in wooden towers resembling old-fashioned library card catalog holders. I'd bought the towers years before because they reminded me of one of my favorite places— the Philadelphia Free

Library on the Parkway. My friends and I would stop at that imposing edifice on our way home from Masterman Junior High school at 17th and Spring Garden. I loved going to that library to search through the card catalogs for the right book to inspire a research project or book report. I was only twelve or thirteen years old then. I had no idea what the future held for me. Now I searched through my wooden CD holders looking for music to inspire my life.

One summer morning, I flipped through my CDs convinced that nothing in my collection could make me feel better. I passed over many of my old standbys dismissively—Nancy Wilson and Cannonball Adderley, Flora Purim, Pharoah Sanders, Doug and Jean Carne, Gary Bartz. What's happening to me? Those were my favorites. I'd lost my kidneys. Was I losing my emotional connection to my favorite music? Feeling low, I decided to leave my CDs alone for a while and listen to the news. Maybe something interesting was happening in the real world. As I closed the CD drawer, my eye caught the spine of a disk I'd overlooked: *Young Disciples/Road to Freedom*. I hadn't played this in months. How'd I overlook this one? Rob gave me the CD last year when he thought I needed uplifting. He was right. I loved every song on the recording. I pulled out the disk and stared at the jacket, remembering that I not only loved the music, but the cover picture also. The photo of the three "young disciples" looking cool and defiant, reminded me of my son and some of his friends.

I slipped the disk into the machine and before I could brace myself, the music oozed out of the speakers. My blood warmed, and I sank into a chair to listen. I stopped the CD and repeated that first song at least five times. Initially, I thought my obsession was with the lead singer, Carleen Anderson's, urgent, compelling contralto. Slowly, I realized that the song's potent refrain was lodged firmly in my head. Those Young Disciples were speaking directly to me with the song "Get Yourself Together." I had to try.

Chapter Eight:
HAPPINESS IS A MAN CALLED JOE

A warm, late September breeze blew across the living room as Bobby Watson's alto flowed melodically from the speakers. After running a few Saturday morning errands, I'd been lying on the sofa all afternoon glued to the Sunday *New York Times Magazine*. Bobby's beautiful horn only perpetuated my lazy mood. He had a sound like no other.

The clanging telephone rudely interrupted my reverie. Who would dare intrude on my splendid Saturday afternoon? Should I get up and answer the phone?

For some inexplicable reason, I decided that I should. I sat up and reached over to the kitchen counter to pick up the receiver. Well, what do you know? I recognized the number.

"Hello," I said. My "hello" sounded like a question rather than a greeting.

"Hey Dine, it's Joe. How you doing?"

That voice. What is it about this man's voice that made me quiver—even after such a long time?

"Hey, Joe. It's been a while," I said trying to sound casual.

"I know, I know," Joe responded, laughing. "You could call me too, you know."

Conversation between Joe and me could be like a chess

match, with each of us carefully choosing the next verbal move before we spoke. Our "game" could go on for a while until one of us gave in and decided to get real. Our conversation was about to get very real.

"Yeah, Joe, that's true, I could call, but I've been busy." What an understatement. Kidney failure, dialysis, a transplant, recovery. Yep, I'd been busy all right.

I couldn't remember the last time I'd spoken with Joe, let alone seen him. Had we spoken in a year? How much did he know about my situation?

Our relationship had always been on, then off, then on again. Sometimes I wondered whether I should call what we had a "relationship." For close to a decade, we'd been basically "hooking up" whenever he was in Philly, or I was in DC. We'd never made any kind of commitment to each other.

Joe Davidson and I went back a long way…back to the 1970s when I was with my ex, Alexs, and Joe was married. I'd heard about Joe before I ever met him. He was something of a legend in Philadelphia's Black progressive circles—a journalist, a founder of the National Association of Black Journalists, a family man, and an all-around "righteous brother."

In those days, all the politically oriented Black people in Philly knew or knew of each other. I may have even caught a glimpse of Joe at a party or two. Still, we wouldn't formally meet until the mid-1980s when I went to a gathering at a mutual friend's house. Joe was there to speak about covering the anti-apartheid movement in South Africa. I was attracted to him at once—he was smart, cute, accomplished, and earnest—exactly my type. Since he was married, we became friends, talking by phone and meeting for dinner on occasion.

When Joe's marriage ended in the early 1990's, we became

more than friends, although life got in the way of us becoming a real couple. At least that's what we told each other. Joe had moved to DC, while I was still in Philly. He had joint custody of his teenage sons, who were his priority. My son, Rob, no longer lived with me but was still a huge part of my life. Joe took on even more family responsibility when he brought his elderly mother from Detroit to live with him in 1994. On top of all these obligations, we both had challenging, time-consuming careers.

I'd always wanted more with Joe. I'd readily make room for him in my life if I thought he felt the same way about me. But over the years, Joe showed me repeatedly that he wasn't available, physically, or emotionally.

"I better guard my heart," I told myself as I stared at the telephone.

Joe's voice brought me back to our conversation. "What's been keeping you so busy?"

Here goes, I thought. I guess I'll find out how much he knows or wants to know.

"I had a kidney transplant," I said, as plain as day. For a few seconds, Joe was silent. I couldn't even hear him breathing. I guess he hadn't known anything.

"What did you say?" He sounded stunned. "Dine, what the hell? When did all this happen?"

Where do I start? One part of me was frustrated and angry with Joe. If he'd stayed in touch, he'd know what was going on. On the other hand, Joe and I had been involved for years and I never once mentioned to him that I had kidney disease. What's more, about the transplant, he was right. I also could have picked up the phone.

I flopped back into the sofa cushions and started my "kidney" story from the top. Joe and I talked for more than an hour, with him stopping me every few minutes to ask for details and clarification. He was a journalist and wanted the details of any story, not only mine. I told him everything.

"Dine, I'm so sorry you've had to go through all this," he said, sounding as emotional as I'd ever heard him. "Was surgery the only solution? Did you try changing your diet, natural or alternative medicine? A transplant seems so drastic."

I found Joe's comments annoying. I hated it when people second-guessed me about the transplant surgery. Didn't he think I knew a transplant was drastic? Did he think I had any other choice?

"Believe me, Joe, the transplant was my only choice. I tried a bunch of other remedies. Nothing made any difference. Once your kidneys start acting up, there's little that can be done to reverse the damage."

"I'm really sorry, Dine. How are you now? Are you in any pain?"

I'd spent enough time with Joe to know he hated pain—his own or anyone else's. *I don't understand why people have to suffer pain,* he'd lament, a sentiment I found innocent and sweet. In my experience, pain was part of life.

"I'm not in pain, Joe, not physical pain anyway. I'm still stunned by what I've been through, but I'm not in pain. The surgery was back in March. I went back to work a few weeks ago—three days a week. I'm taking good care of myself."

"I want to come up and see you. Maybe I can help out—take you grocery shopping or something."

Another silence fell between us. I was searching my heart and mind for the right response. This was a moment of truth. I'd love to have Joe around. At the same time, I knew I wasn't ready for the "on again, off again" that came with Joe Davidson. I was still too raw and vulnerable from my ordeal. I knew from experience Joe would be non-committal. I'd be "cruisin' for a bruisin'."

"I don't think you coming up here's a good idea, Joe."

Once I said those words, I wanted to reach into the air, grab them, and throw them right back down my throat. But I knew I was right.

"Why not?" Joe asked, sounding surprised and hurt.

Why not? How do I answer that question? Let's see… You coming up is not a good idea because I'm too needy right now? Because I know you'll let me down in the end; because I won't want you to leave. Any of these answers would have been true, but I blurted out a response I knew he would understand clearly.

"Joe, I'm seeing someone."

I couldn't believe I'd said that. I didn't want to hurt Joe, but I told the truth. I was seeing someone. My friend Ed had been a fixture in my life since before the surgery. He'd taken me to dialysis and doctors' appointments, run errands for me, and been around when I needed a man's company. I knew Ed wasn't the man I wanted to be with forever, but I could depend on him right now. I wasn't sure I could depend on Joe. He might break my heart and I'd already lost one body part.

"So, this relationship is serious?" Joe asked, his voice almost cracking at the end of his question.

"For now."

"Wow," Joe said, as he let out a long, loud sigh. "I hope you're going to be okay."

"I'll be okay," I answered, although I wasn't at all sure about that.

"Well, let's at least stay in touch."

"Of course," I murmured, but I didn't expect to hear from Joe any time soon. I probably wouldn't call him either. Then, our conversation was over.

Shit, I thought. Have I made the biggest mistake of my life? After sitting on the couch with that question for a few minutes, I answered myself. *No, you didn't make a mistake. You must take care of yourself, even if it hurts. Taking care of yourself is your main job.*

∼

BY SEPTEMBER, 2000, after six months of medical leave, I still didn't feel strong enough—mentally or physically—to return to work full time. After talking with my boss, who was the president of the company I worked for, we decided that I'd come back only three days a week (Tuesday, Wednesday, and Thursday) until the end of the year and return to my job full-time in January, 2001. I'd be paid a part-time salary, but I'd done the math and decided that I could handle the pay cut.

I don't know exactly why my boss agreed to this arrangement. I was good at my job but certainly not indispensable. All I could do was accept my good fortune and be grateful. This schedule would give me extended weekends to continue my recovery. I knew that not everyone who went through a trauma could take the time they needed to recover without having to worry about how they would eat, take care of their children, or pay the rent. Sometimes, I thought about my days not so long ago in ratty apartments and living on welfare and food stamps. I'd worked hard for my advantages. Still, I reminded myself often to be grateful.

Once back on the job, I saw that my long absence had not been without consequences. I'd been moved to a smaller office without notification, my assistant had taken a job with another company, and my assignments had been divided up among colleagues. Not surprisingly, the company had developed new projects and priorities while I was out. I still carried the title of executive vice president, but I was out of the loop.

At first, I resented these changes and felt a bit paranoid. Is this my boss' way of getting back at me for taking so much time off? I contemplated looking for another position in the social policy field but didn't yet have the energy for a job search. I needed to make the current situation work for me, at least until I could figure out my next steps. When my boss suggested that I help develop a few new "special projects" that had come into the company, I was ecstatic. Ha, I laughed at myself. Not long ago I would have shuddered at the thought of such an assignment with the dreaded "special projects" title, where irrelevant executives go to die. However, the position gave me plenty of independence and limited the amount of travel I was expected to do. Since I was primarily working alone, I had the liberty to work at home or in the office—the perfect situation for me.

With my work life more or less under control, I did my best to start rebuilding my social life, resuming my involvement with a few arts organizations, and hanging out with close friends. Thankfully, no one seemed very interested in talking about my transplant experience, including me. I sensed that the subject of "transplants" was too scary for most people. After quick exchanges about my health and comments about me "looking great," people seemed happy to move on. I was too.

Fortunately for me, Ed was still in my corner. I knew he wasn't a long-term partner. We weren't, as I'd heard older Black folks say, "equally yoked," a term that I'm told can be found somewhere in the Bible. In other words, we weren't on the same level as far as education and income are concerned. I was born poor, but now I had a master's degree, a professional job, and a downtown condo. He was a broke, street-smart jazz musician and recovering heroin addict. In theory, I'd always thought these kinds of differences shouldn't matter, but I'd found out that in real life, they can. Frankly, I was an "uptown" girl, and he was a "downtown" guy, to put things roughly. We had vastly different approaches to life and our disagreements were deep and many. Nevertheless, we could lie on the couch and listen to Miles Davis and Shirley Horn for hours without saying a word. What's more, Ed had been by my side during the whole transplant business. And he thought I was perfect, even with my jury-rigged body. That kind of connection and acceptance was priceless to me.

Despite my progress re-entering the world, on some days I still felt like Humpty Dumpty after a great fall. Why did I need someone else's kidney? Is this all real? Am I dreaming? Seeing the enormous tray of pills sitting on my kitchen counter was always a stark reminder that I was, indeed, wide awake.

One morning I decided to act on something I'd been thinking about ever since the surgery. I made an appointment to see a therapist. I wanted to talk with someone besides the kidney doctors, who only seemed interested in whether my new kidney was working.

"Black people don't go to therapy" is a common narrative. However, that wasn't true for me. I'd had my first stint with counseling in the early 1980s when I was living in the Twin Cities. At the encouragement of my friend Kathleen, I joined a women's therapy circle to try and keep my bearings as my second marriage disintegrated. In all honesty, I also knew I needed to address what seemed like the never-ending cycle of sadness and anger that had haunted me my entire life, including my distant relationship with my family, especially my father, and my dysfunctional marriages. In this therapy group, I learned about owning my own "stuff" and confronting people who mistreated me. However, I was the only Black woman in the circle, not surprising, since in those days, the Black population of the Twin Cities was less than five percent. I stayed in the group because I was lost and vulnerable and needed a sense of belonging. But there were times when I felt that the group's therapists and most of the other group members had no meaningful knowledge of who I was or where I'd come from.

This time around I chose Lydia Richards. I simply asked people I knew about a Black female therapist and her name surfaced several times. I'll never forget the first day I walked into her tiny office in a nondescript business complex in West Philly. I took one look at her—a short, chubby, timid-looking woman, and immediately felt disheartened. Had I made a mistake? Something about this woman's appearance didn't inspire my confidence.

Richards stood up from her desk and extended her hand to me. "Bernardine," she asked sweetly, "How can I help you?"

Richards' voice sounded like a bird. Her speech sounded more like chirping than talking. But she radiated warmth and kindness that I felt right away. Before I could answer her, I surprised myself by bursting into tears.

How could she help me? Where should I begin: With the still wounded little girl whose father could be brutal? With the woman who'd racked up two divorces by the time she was thirty-nine? With my confused feelings about having to accept a kidney from my older sister? With my near "freak out" after my transplant surgery? With my quiet fear about the FSGS returning?

Richards quickly enveloped me in a comforting hug. She patted my arm and guided me to a chair.

"Bernardine," she chirped, "I see the pain you're in and I'm sure you have every right to be in pain, but believe me, you're going to be okay. Please, sit down."

Richards handed me a tissue from a box on her desk.

"Here, blow your nose," she said sympathetically. She stood patiently beside the chair, handing me tissue after tissue as tears continued to flood my face. Part of me felt embarrassed at my display, but another part of me knew that I wasn't the first person to have a good cry in her office. That's why she kept a big box of tissues sitting on her desk.

Because of my flexible work schedule and ability to work from home, I saw Richards every Friday from 1:00-2:00 for two years. While I guess that she was about my age, I thought of her as a wise, compassionate, but no-nonsense aunt. The fact that she was Black meant a great deal to me. We were "tribe," as the saying goes. She was Black and female in America, like me. I trusted her.

While Richards was clear that she couldn't and wouldn't try to solve all my problems, she encouraged me to consider my issues and fears in a different light. She saw that my tears and sadness were not only about my kidney transplant but an accumulation of disappointments.

My Father: "Yes, your father was an angry man who took his anger out on you inappropriately. But anger is what your father knew. You've told me that your dad's father left the family when your dad was just a child and that his mother—your grandmother, was a tough, angry woman. I know you might not want to hear this, but your father, Bernard, did the best he could, given what he had to work with. Now, you have to decide if you want to carry that same anger around or if you want to let it go."

My divorces: "How old were you when you got married the first time? Nineteen? Twenty? You and your son's father were so young. What did you know about marriage? Did you see many examples of good marriages when you were growing up? And don't be so hard on yourself about the second marriage. Sweetheart, you were looking for love and found that relationships take more than love. Give yourself a break. Learn to love and value yourself. From what I can see you're an amazing person. Look at all you've been through, all you've accomplished. Real love will come when you're ready for it."

My kidney surgery and receiving a kidney from my sister: "Bernardine, you've had to carry a lot in your life. I'm glad you reacted emotionally after your surgery. A kidney transplant is huge. I'd rather see you 'freak out,' as you call it, than act like nothing happened. You made an excellent decision to give yourself lots of time to heal before going back to work. You're still healing, but you're taking care of yourself. I'm not worried about you. You'll be okay. As for your sister, clearly, she loves you and thinks you're worthy or she wouldn't have given you her kidney. Now you need to allow yourself to feel worthy and fully accept her gift. You must accept that you needed someone, and she came through for you. This time you didn't have to take care of yourself. Your sister took care of you. Accept it."

When I told Richards that I felt guilty about not calling my sister after the surgery, she also gave me a perspective that surprised me and eased my mind.

"Your sister hasn't been in touch with you much, either, right? She may have some unresolved feelings about being your donor and needs time to herself also. You're both healing. Don't worry. You'll be in touch when the time is right. If you have issues to work on, you can take care of them then."

As for my fears about the future and the possible recurrence of the FSGS, Richards said, "Take care of yourself today. Value yourself now and let the future take its course. If you must face FSGS in the future, you will, and you'll be okay. The disease may rock your world for a moment, but you'll pull yourself together because that's who you are."

Those Fridays with Richards gave me time and space to be vulnerable. On some afternoons, when I couldn't find words to express myself, tears would fall out of my eyes for the entire hour. Other afternoons, words would flow from my mouth like a river of tears. Richards encouraged me to be sad without shame. She'd tell me, "Sadness doesn't make you weak and denying your sadness doesn't make you tough." Her words were a revelation to me. Where I grew up, people showed their anger all the time, but rarely their sadness. I could count the good cries I'd had as an adult. Growing up, if I looked like I was going to cry without what seemed like a good enough reason, some adult would threaten to "give me something to cry about."

As the year 2000 became 2001, I realized that I'd survived my personal apocalypse. March 3 would mark the first anniversary of the transplant surgery. Surprising myself, one January day, I called Baby Alice. We still didn't talk that often, but that day I felt a deep need to connect with her.

"Thank you so much for taking such good care of me before the surgery and for saving my life." I'd thanked Baby Alice many times before, but I still felt that I couldn't thank her enough.

"What's the matter?" my sister asked, sounding alarmed. "Is everything okay?"

"Yeah, Sis, I'm fine. I wanted to say hi and thank you again."

"Well, you can stop thanking me," she said, nonchalantly. "I'd do it all again if I could. God gave us two kidneys, so we could give one to someone in need. You needed a kidney, and I gave you one of mine. I believe that's what God wanted me to do."

I closed my eyes, listening to my sister and wondered if she had any fear or uncertainty at all about having her kidney removed. Did her religion make her fearless? I didn't know, but as my therapist suggested, I would have to take my sister's word that she was telling me her truth.

"Well, Sis," I said, "I sure hope I won't need another kidney, so let's not even go there." Quickly, I changed the subject.

"Do you realize we have an anniversary coming up?"

"Of course, I do," Alice responded. "March 3rd."

I couldn't believe my ears when I heard my voice say, "Let's have a party and celebrate. We can gather at Mommy's house. I'll make an invitation and we'll invite all our family and friends, so everyone can see we're both doing well."

I hung up the phone with Baby Alice, in disbelief. Had I proposed a party? Was I going to stand around in my parents' living room laughing and grinning with people about something I'd hardly spoken about for fifteen years? What had gotten into me? Relief? Growing confidence about my life? I didn't know but decided to go with it.

I designed the invitation from a piece of clip art I found online—a silhouette of two little Black girls, one slightly taller than the other, holding hands as they skipped down the street. More than fifty people crowded into my parents' house to laugh, eat, hug Baby Alice and me, and tell us how great we looked. More than once, I heard a family member comment, "Bernard would be so proud of you two, taking care of each other like this." Even Mommy was smiling. So was I.

WITH ONE YEAR of living with a transplanted kidney behind me, I began to think that maybe I had a good life ahead. I still had bad days and couldn't pass a mirror without scowling at my Prednisone-induced puffy face. But at least I was asking myself the right question: Can I get on with my life now?

One evening when I was feeling particularly lonely, I decided to call Joe Davidson's number. No matter what was going on with me, Joe was always on my mind. We hadn't spoken for about a year after I'd told him not to visit me in Philly. The day after that conversation he'd sent me an email with the word "cliff" in the subject line. While I was pleased to see a message from him, I couldn't imagine what "cliff" could be about. Who in the world is "Cliff," I wondered? I don't recall the exact wording of Joe's note, but the bottom line of his message was that he was shocked and hurt by my request that he not visit me. He felt I had dropped him from a "cliff."

My mouth fell open in stunned disbelief as I read Joe's note. "What the hell are you talking about?" I shouted at the computer screen as if I were shouting at Joe himself. Then I spent the next five minutes bawling him out in my mind: So, you feel like you've been dropped from a cliff? Since when have you taken our relationship seriously? I didn't know if I could depend on you. That's why I asked you not to come up. Damn you, Joe.

Once I'd finished fuming, I realized there was a hopeful sign in Joe's note. Maybe the idea that I was seeing someone else had shaken him. I wrestled with whether to answer him and finally responded with this one line of truth.

"Joe, I had no idea." He never responded, and I decided to leave him alone. My life was complicated enough.

However, a year had passed since Joe's "cliff" note. I'm not looking for complications, I reasoned as I dialed. I wanted to say hello and see how he was doing. My hands shook a bit. Must be the Prednisone, I laughed. I still knew his number by heart.

The telephone rang three or four times. I was ready to hang up when I heard him say hello. I knew Joe. Something was wrong. He didn't seem to have much energy. This was not the Joe I knew. Please. Don't let anything be wrong with this man.

"Hey, Joe," I said. "What's the matter?"

For a moment there was silence on the line. Didn't he know who I was? Didn't my number come up on his caller ID? Don't tell me he's forgotten my number, or worse, my voice.

"Oh, hi, Dine," Joe responded finally, sounding a bit more like himself. Still, I could tell something was wrong.

"What's going on, Joe?" I asked. "You sound strange."

At first, there was silence again, then I heard a sigh.

"My mom died last month."

This time I was silent. Tears welled in my eyes. I'd never met Margaret Gretchen Davidson, but Joe talked to me about her often. He was an only child and very close to his mother. He adored her. Based on Joe's description, I had a picture of Mrs. Davidson in my head. She was tall, fair, reserved, classy, and beautiful.

"I'm so sorry. Why didn't you let me know?"

Joe sighed again.

"Oh, Dine," he said, his voice still low. "I'm sorry. There was so much to do, and I had to handle most of the arrangements myself. I tried to get notices out to as many people as possible, but I'm sure I missed some people…" His voice trailed off.

"Joe, I'm so sorry," I repeated, this time more emphatically. "I would have come down," I said without thinking. The truth is, I would have gone down to DC in a flash to do whatever I could to help him.

"Dine, I appreciate that, but my mother's services were in Detroit. That's where her life was. She'd been in DC with me for seven years, but she was never at home here. I wouldn't expect you to come to Detroit."

"No," I said, "but I could have come down to DC to be with you, to do what I could to help. How are you doing?"

"I'm okay," he said half-heartedly, "but it's been hard, Dine. When Mom died, I was out in California with my cousin Alan. I'd taken her to one of those short-term senior care facilities for a few days, so I could get a break. She hated those places and honestly, I hated taking her to them, but I needed some time away. Alan and I were driving along the coast in his convertible when I got the call that she was gone." Joe's voice cracked. I felt my heart break for him.

"Can I do anything for you?" I asked, fully aware that, not too long ago, I had denied Joe the opportunity to support me during a tough time.

"No thank you," he responded, politely. "I'll be okay. I'm out on my back porch looking at the trees and listening to the birds. My Mom loved sitting out here."

"Joe, please call me if you need anything," I pleaded. "I can take the train and come down to DC easily."

"Sure, I will," he said. "How are you doing? I'm sorry I didn't ask earlier. How's your health?" Joe's tone was very apologetic. He prided himself on being polite.

"I'm well Joe, feeling better all the time. Don't worry about me. Take care of yourself."

Before we hung up, I promised Joe that I'd call the next time I was in DC. "Maybe we can have dinner or a drink."

"I'd like that," Joe said, sounding like he might want to see me. "Hopefully, I'll be better company by then."

During that conversation, I felt a subtle shift between Joe and me. He seemed more open to me. What am I sensing? I asked myself. Could there be a chance for something more between us? Or is he feeling vulnerable right now, caught up in the sadness of his mother's death? I warned myself not to get too carried away.

I took my own advice and didn't make any moves. With Joe grieving and me just getting my act together, this was probably not a great time to jump into anything. However, Joe and I stayed in touch more regularly. Like two good friends, we'd check on each other once a month or so, to see how the other was recovering from life's wounds. We seemed to be getting closer. But I wanted to see Joe in person. I needed to know if I was imagining this increased "closeness."

In February 2002, I had the opportunity to attend a conference in DC. I can't recall the subject of the meeting, but I'll never forget the dinner Joe and I had at Equinox Restaurant, just off Farragut Square. As we talked, I thought, no, I'm not imagining anything. What a sweet evening. When we left the restaurant, I didn't invite Joe back to my hotel room, as I'd done many times in the past, and he didn't ask.

"Do you want me to hail a cab for you?" he asked. "I'd walk you back to your hotel, but it might be too cold for you," he said, laughing. "I'm from Michigan. I can take this wind."

I laughed too. "Yes, a cab will do just fine." We'd known each other long enough to have a few jokes between us. Joe would walk anywhere in any kind of weather. He thought I was much too sensitive to the elements.

A taxi pulled up in front of us before we were ready to say goodbye. As Joe opened the door for me, I kissed him on the cheek and said, "Something's changed between us." Joe kissed me back and said, "Sometimes things need to change."

Back home in Philadelphia, I couldn't help thinking that something had finally started between me and Joe. Something real.

∼

NEITHER JOE NOR I wanted to rush into anything. I didn't make any plans for another "business" trip to DC, and Joe didn't immediately head north on I-95 to visit me. I told myself that we should let our relationship unfold slowly. Joe and I stayed in touch, however, with long, sometimes serious, sometimes funny, sometimes sexy, telephone conversations. He was finally letting me in.

"What's changed between us?" I boldly asked him one night during one of our marathon phone sessions. As soon as I'd asked the question, I wanted to take the words back. We were growing closer, but Joe still wasn't the kind of guy to pour his heart out. However, he answered me with a level of detail I didn't expect.

"Dine, my feelings toward you haven't changed. I've always wanted to see more of you but couldn't. First, there's the distance. Philly is what I call a "middle distance" away from DC —too far to get to as much as you'd like, but close enough to think you can get there more often than you can. In a "middle distance" relationship, someone is always going to be disappointed. Know what I mean?"

Hmm. I needed to think about that one. "Middle distance" sounded like gibberish to me.

"Really, Joe? I never thought distance was our problem. I think the problem's been commitment. Maybe we haven't been ready."

"Well, that's my second point," Joe said, his voice rising slightly. "I haven't been ready."

I kept my mouth shut and let him keep talking. He hadn't been ready? What an understatement.

"I admit, I've had a lot on my plate for a long time now," Joe continued. "My mom needed a lot of care. That's why I brought her to DC from Detroit to live with me. I also had my boys—Hakimu and Jasiri. My ex-wife and I had joint custody, but after the boys started high school, they both stopped going to their mom's house and stayed with me. Now my mom's gone, Hakimu is off to college, and Jasiri, well, he'll be off to school soon too. Now, I feel like I'm ready for a relationship."

I heard myself gasp for air. I'd been listening to Joe so intently that I'd forgotten to breathe. But there was one question.

"With me?" I asked. "Are you ready for a relationship with me?"

Joe laughed as if he thought my question was silly. "Well, I'd like to try."

With those words, Joe and I began seeing much more of each other. The "middle distance" between Philly and DC was still something of an obstacle, but we managed to make the most of our time together. One of the most memorable dates in our renewed relationship was a camping trip we took. Neither of us can remember the location of the campsite.

Early in May, 2002, while he was traveling in South Africa with his sons, Joe invited me, by email, to an annual Memorial Day weekend camping trip he took with a group of journalists and other Black professionals. The group called themselves

"Black Pack," which I thought was very cool. Included with the invitation was an extensive list of equipment and provisions (including a tent and sleeping bags) that, if I were interested in going with him on the trip, I'd have to pick up at an REI store outside of Philadelphia. Joe was in South Africa and wouldn't be home in time to pull all the camping gear together. While he denies it, I'm convinced that this assignment from him was a test designed to determine my "outdoors quotient." Joe is an Eagle Scout and avid camper. If I couldn't organize a camping weekend, maybe I wasn't "the one."

I'll be the first to admit that I'm mostly a city girl, but I was determined to ace Joe's test—and I did. Our Memorial Day weekend was an excellent adventure, including a colossal thunderstorm on Saturday night that forced us to huddle closely in our zip-together sleeping bags. By the time our camping weekend was over, I knew I was falling deeply in love with Joe. Friends teased that any man who could get me to sleep in a tent in the woods had to be special. I assured them that he was.

A key question, though: was Joe falling in love with me? I knew he cared about me. But I wasn't sure how deeply his feelings ran. I was encouraged, however, when we agreed to disentangle ourselves from any other "romantic" attachments. This meant saying goodbye to my friend Ed. We hadn't been seeing much of each other, but I needed to let him know that our relationship—at least in the "carnal" sense, was over. I took no pleasure in that task. Ed had been in my corner through tough times when Joe wasn't there. But my relationship with Joe had real potential. As I'd always known, my relationship with Ed did not.

A few weeks later, in June, Joe asked me to attend a friend's wedding with him on the beautiful island of Anguilla, West Indies. This social occasion was much more in my lane than a camping trip. Without a second thought, I took a week of vacation days and met him there. Until I reached Anguilla, I didn't realize how much I needed that trip. The lush island surroundings and the beautiful wedding, with all the guests dressed in white, was a balm for my spirit. One night as we lay in bed listening to the ocean lap against the beach, Joe whispered "I love you" into my ear. I was so shocked I could not speak for a moment.

"I never thought I'd hear those words from you," I said finally. "I love you too."

For the first time in years, I was happy. Joe Davidson loved me. That fact alone made life instantly better. My therapist, Lydia Richards, had assured me that "real love would come when I was ready for it," and she'd been right. More of the strength and confidence I'd lost during my illness began to return. Once I allowed myself to believe in Joe's love for me, living with a kidney transplant began to feel almost routine. Yes, I had to take tons of medicine, but now I found myself gulping the pills down without much thought and sometimes without water. Yes, I still felt the side effects of the Prednisone and the other immunosuppressants, like shaking hands and anxiety, but I was learning to talk myself through these episodes. Yes, I was still annoyed by my "chipmunk" cheeks. However, Joe didn't seem to notice them or better yet, thought I was "fine" anyway. I'd gone through a big trauma, but two years later, I was still standing, and Joe Davidson was standing beside me.

Could the sun finally be shining on me? In addition to being in love, my health was surprisingly good. My creatinine level was stable and in the "good" range…not perfect, but good. As Dr. Rudnick would say, "We're not going for perfect. Good is good enough."

What's more, work was still going well. I delivered on my "special project" assignments and my boss left me to myself. I worked at home as much as I liked, coming into the office only when necessary. Sometimes I missed the "hubbub" of office life and the power trip that came from being a leader in the company. But I told myself that I'd needed a slower pace for a long time, even before the transplant.

Suddenly, out of what felt like nowhere, fate clocked me with a one-two punch. First, in October, I lost my job. I would have seen this first hit coming had I been paying attention. The economy had been in trouble since 2000, with the dramatic deflation of the dot-com bubble. By 2002, the stock market was in sharp decline. The nonprofit research company I worked for received most of its funding from large foundations that took big losses from that fall. On occasion, when I was in the office, I'd heard whispers about layoffs. Still, I was blindsided when I was among those given the unwelcome news. One afternoon, after letting me blab on with an update on my projects, my boss said, "Dine, I'm sorry to tell you that we have to let you go. The Hewlett Foundation cut funding for your work."

Stunned, I thought, me? You're letting me go? After fourteen years? I'm the only Black executive in this place. I thought I and my projects were "special." Although I was close to tears, I refused to cry in this man's presence. I gathered my papers and myself and left the office that same day. I didn't even bother to take the company up on their offer of office space until my last day.

After the shock of my dismissal wore off, I came to my senses and saw things more clearly. My insistence on taking an extended disability leave and my disengagement from office life once I returned was probably as much a reason for my being laid off as the economy. I'd been foolish to think I wouldn't pay for those decisions.

Still, I was fortunate. Because of my executive position and lengthy tenure, I left the company with a more than adequate severance package, the company's agreement to support my unemployment claim, and my laptop. The layoff also prompted me to start the social policy consulting practice I'd always considered. While my boss sent a few job possibilities my way, I had no desire at that moment to go work for another company. My research, writing, and management skills were widely known in the policy field, and I didn't think I'd have any trouble generating clients. A few months after losing my job, I had enough consulting work to support myself through 2003, including a major assignment from the employer that had just laid me off.

Supporting myself, however, wasn't my immediate problem. The second blow to hit me landed in the early spring of 2003 and ripped away my optimism about the future. I'd hardly settled into a chair in his examining room for my quarterly checkup when Rudnick broke this news to me. "Ms. Watson, your last labs showed a small amount of blood and protein in your urine and your creatinine has ticked up a bit."

Rudnick paused and stared down at me over his glasses. He seemed to be waiting for my response. I had none. I was having trouble understanding him. What the hell was he talking about? As he started to speak again, I began to understand what he was saying. My insides began to shake.

"…These symptoms could be signs of your body rejecting the transplant or recurrence of the FSGS, I'm not sure yet. I'm going to increase the Vasotec to try and reduce the amount of protein in your urine as we tried before the transplant. Maybe we'll have better results with the new kidney. I also want to get you in here for a biopsy, so we can see what's going on in that transplanted kidney. And we'll make an appointment for you in urology to see if we can find out where that blood's coming from."

All I could do was sink down into the hard plastic chair. How could this be happening to me again? I hadn't noticed a thing. No, I hadn't been weighing myself weekly like I was supposed to. No, I hadn't been taking my blood pressure daily like I was supposed to. But I had been taking my medicine religiously and feeling fine. Happy, even. Am I never supposed to be happy?

Later, when I recounted the news to Joe in a telephone conversation, he was philosophical.

"Rudnick says the Vasotec could have good results, right? Why don't you wait until you do all the stuff he says before you start to worry? Didn't the transplant surgeons say that these rejection episodes might happen?"

I loved Joe and valued his opinion, but his calm tone made me angry. I responded impatiently.

"Yes, yes, I know, Joe. But Rudnick also said that my symptoms could be signs of the FSGS coming back. I've been through all this before Joe—the protein in my urine, rising creatinine… and the Vasotec? The miracle drug? We tried that before, Joe, back when you weren't around. It didn't work. I went through all that by myself."

I knew I'd taken a swipe at Joe, to remind him of the times when he hadn't been around to support me in my illness. All I wanted to do was lash out at anyone or blame someone, even Joe, for my predicament. So, I kept talking, until I could hear my voice dropping to a low, angry growl.

"Joe, you don't know what you're talking about, and you don't know how I feel. This is my life that's on the line. You don't know how many times Rudnick told me that nephrologists don't know how to fix this kidney disease. At a certain point, the only treatments left are transplants and dialysis. I've already tried both. What happens now?"

"You do what Rudnick suggests."

Joe's tone made me so angry I wanted to scream. But honestly, I didn't know who I was angry with—Joe, Rudnick, the whole goddamn universe?

∼

THE RESULTS of the biopsy were inconclusive.

"From the specimen we took, we couldn't see whether there's additional scarring in the new kidney," Rudnick said. "We could go back in to retrieve more tissue, but I wouldn't suggest that. We could end up injuring the kidney or introducing infection."

No, no, no, I screamed inside my head. My body had already been cut open too many times. Besides, if the tissue from my new kidney showed scarring, could the doctors do anything about it?

The following week, I gritted my teeth and went through with the urological exam. I asked Rudnick to explain the procedure to me in detail. When he told me that I would be sedated so that the urologist could easily stick a scope into my bladder and look around, I asked my sister Linda to come along with me. I was surprised at how relieved I was to see her in the lobby of the hospital on the day of the test, and even more thankful when afterward, she helped me into a taxi before going off to work.

The exam itself was an unpleasant piece of business, but inconclusive also.

"The good news is," Rudnick said, "the blood's not coming from your transplant. On the other hand," he said with a frown, "we can't tell where the blood is coming from. The bleeding could be something to worry about or not. I suggest we not worry about the bleeding unless it gets worse. Let's focus on upping the Vasotec. With any luck, we can lessen or even eliminate the protein in your urine."

Exhausted and scared, I responded to Rudnick with a snotty question. "So, we're relying on luck now?" I asked.

Rudnick's modest reply surprised me. "I'll take all the luck I can get."

∽

The summer of 2003 was a roller coaster. Dr. Rudnick increased my Vasotec dose, and initially, the amount of protein in my urine decreased.

"Vasotec is a great drug," he'd declare. In response, I'd exhale and dance, high on relief and happiness. But the good results wouldn't last long. In a month or so, the protein would reappear in my urine and my spirits would plunge. Rudnick tried various doses and combinations of medications designed to control my blood pressure, reduce the protein in my urine, and protect my kidney function. The results were disappointing. A new strategy would work for a while, but in the end, neither luck nor medical science seemed to be on my side.

Finally, Rudnick concluded, "We'll have to do our best to preserve as much of your kidney function as we can, for as long as we can. That's all we can do now."

I was stunned and devastated. I hadn't expected this news three and one-half years into my transplant, especially since my donor, my sister Alice, and I were a perfect blood and tissue match. I could still hear the doctors telling me, "A living related donor gives you the best chance of success. Your new kidney should last at least twenty years."

Again, I retreated into my old friend, secrecy No one, besides Joe and my doctors—not Baby Alice, my mother, or my son, Robert—knew the trouble I was in. Fortunately, Joe was right by my side throughout all the wicked ups and downs. The "middle distance" between us ceased to be a problem. On Fridays, he'd jump in his car and speed up I-95 to my place for the weekend. As a consultant, all I needed was my laptop and cellphone to spend days at a time at his house in DC.

One evening as we sat curled up on the sofa at my apartment staring out of the window as cars flew across the blue bridge, I fell into a particularly melancholy mood. "You know what scares me more than dealing with kidney failure again?"

Joe looked at me and said, "Where did that thought come from?"

"I'm scared to be sick and not able to take care of myself. I'm okay now because I have work and can afford to pay my insurance premiums. What if I have a lull in work assignments? The premiums I pay as an independent consultant are astronomical."

Joe stared at me intently for a moment and then said, "I have insurance."

I tried my best to keep my cool and not fall off the sofa.

"What's that supposed to mean? Was that a proposal?" I looked up at him wide-eyed.

"Sure," he answered, with a grin and a shrug.

Despite his nonchalance, I knew Joe was serious. He wouldn't play with a subject like marriage. I didn't say another word, but let the moment hang in the air while we snuggled even closer.

Life continued as usual for several months after that evening on my sofa, except that Joe and I grew closer every day. Only our children and a few close friends were aware of our intention to marry. One day as we talked with a close friend about my traveling to San Francisco for a business meeting, she piped up and said, "Why don't you get married out there? You'll be close to Reno or Lake Tahoe."

Joe and I both laughed at that idea. However, a few days later, during one of our regular evening calls, Joe said in a wistful tone, "I've always wanted to see Lake Tahoe."

I followed his comment with a wistful remark of my own. "And I've always wanted a proper proposal."

On April 15, 2004, Joe surprised me with his version of a "proper" proposal. While we sat at Blues Alley, DC's famed jazz club, waiting to see saxophonist Kenny Garrett, Joe passed me a napkin on which he'd scrawled, "Will you marry me?" This time I couldn't keep quiet. I said yes.

While I flew out to San Francisco for my business meeting, Joe made all the wedding arrangements, from applying for our wedding license to booking our hotel and wedding site in Incline Village, Lake Tahoe, Nevada. On a lunch break from my meeting, I raced into a nearby Marc Jacobs boutique and bought a dress, shoes, earrings, bag, and wrap. Joe met me at the San Francisco Airport, and we flew off like giggling teens, first to Reno to pick up our license and then to Tahoe. We didn't even have wedding rings yet, but neither of us cared. As I thought back over the tribulations of the past several years of my life, I could hardly believe something so good was happening to me.

BERNARDINE WATSON

On the afternoon of April 25th, Joe and were married by Lake Tahoe under a big tree—just the two of us, a minister he'd found in our hotel services directory, a kindly gentleman from the hotel groundskeeping staff who agreed to be our witness and two wild geese quacking happily in the background.

Chapter Nine:
TRAVELING AND OTHER MERCIES

"I'd suggest you take your trip soon," Dr. Kraus said straightforwardly.

Ed Kraus was my new doctor at Johns Hopkins Hospital in Baltimore, Maryland. Dr. Rudnick had recommended Kraus when I told him I was getting married and moving to DC.

Rudnick seemed taken aback that I was leaving his care at this point in my illness.

"Do you have a nephrologist down there?" he asked quizzically, then adding, "I can't think of anyone in DC specifically, but Ed Kraus at Hopkins in Baltimore is tops in the field."

Dr. Kraus is a slight, wiry man with a high-pitched voice and a habit of waving his arms around wildly when he talks. Both Joe and I liked and trusted him right away. He was forthright, kind, and had a personal touch. But most important, he was a premier nephrologist at Johns Hopkins—the hospital, ranked number #1 in the country by *U. S. News and World Reports* in 2004 and for fourteen years in a row before that. On one of our early visits to his office, we told Kraus about our desire to take a long trip abroad to celebrate our recent marriage.

"Go now while you can," he warned. "Ms. Watson, you'll be on dialysis by the end of the year."

BERNARDINE WATSON

This news was not what we'd driven from DC to Baltimore on a hot August day to hear. Joe had taken yet another day from his job as editor at the Joint Center for Political and Economic Studies. I'd once again put off work on a consulting assignment. We were expecting a more hopeful prognosis.

"I know you're disappointed," he continued sympathetically. "But your test results show no other underlying reason for the spike in your creatinine level but a recurrence of the FSGS in your transplanted kidney."

"Dr. Kraus," I interrupted, finally able to speak the words stuck in my throat, "how can you be sure that I'll be on dialysis in a few months?"

For the first time, I saw a tiny flash of exasperation in Kraus' face, but he recovered quickly and said kindly, "Ms. Watson, I've been treating kidney patients for a long time. I can see kidney failure coming. When you're back from your trip, I want you to see Jack Moore over at Washington Hospital Center. I'll call him. Moore is a former army nephrologist, one of the best—a tough guy, but he takes excellent care of his patients. You need someplace closer to home."

If I hadn't been sitting down, I think I would've toppled right over. I glanced at Joe in the chair beside me. We'd been married for a few months, but at that moment, he looked like he'd aged a few years. I didn't want to kill the man.

Joe and I had been willing to brave interstate traffic between Washington, DC and Baltimore, hoping that a renowned kidney doctor at the famous Johns Hopkins Hospital could bring my dying transplanted kidney back to life. Apparently not. I'd been told many times that FSGS is a real motherfucker. Why had I gotten my hopes up?

We walked out of Hopkins, into the sticky heat and began

the drive home without uttering a word. The car radio was tuned to NPR and story after story about the 2004 presidential election. Ordinarily, Joe and I, both news junkies, prattled back and forth about whatever topic flowed over the air waves, but that day, even a story about Bush and Kerry's slug fest over votes in Ohio, couldn't elicit comment from either of us.

As soon as Joe pulled up in front of our house, I swung around to climb out of the car. I looked down and could see that my feet and ankles were swollen. Ugh. I was retaining fluid, proof that my kidneys were slowing down. I struggled like an old lady to get out of the car.

Finally, I was at our front door. Once inside, I stepped over the pile of mail waiting on the vestibule floor and headed for the stairs, unbuttoning my sweaty clothing as I went. All I wanted to do was go straight to bed and pull the cool sheet up over my head. I heard Joe's footsteps right behind me. Soon, both of us were laying under the top sheet naked.

I don't remember who began to cry first. I hadn't seen or heard Joe cry before and was relieved to see that I'd married a man who would shed tears when warranted. Exhausted, we fell asleep. I woke up to hear Joe blowing his nose in the bathroom. He sounded like a flock of honking geese. Flopping down on his side of the bed, Joe said, "I guess we better start planning that trip."

We both liked to travel and saw this trip as the first of many grand adventures together. After we'd married in April, going away immediately hadn't seemed important. We had a lot to take care of, especially selling my condo in Philly so I could move to DC. We also wanted to wait until after I'd seen Dr. Kraus at Hopkins. Maybe we could fly off on the heels of good news about my health. That certainly hadn't worked out. Now, we needed to get away now more than ever. Whether Kraus' dire prediction was right or not, we needed to escape, relax, and face whatever awaited when we returned.

Joe did all the planning for our trip, as he'd done for our wedding. Because of his work as a journalist and foreign correspondent, Joe was much more adept than I at pouring over flight schedules, finding hotels, and comparing prices. We'd take three weeks to explore Paris, Nice, and Barcelona with an overnight in Madrid, and a day in London on the way home. Joe had plenty of vacation time and my consulting schedule was flexible.

"Let's get lost," we told each other, quoting the title of a favorite jazz standard.

The closer Joe and I came to leaving the country, the more I feared that Kraus could be right in his diagnosis. Increasingly, I was plagued with exhaustion, nausea, indigestion, and diarrhea. Between fluid retention from my decreased kidney function and the effects of Prednisone, I couldn't bear to look at my bloated face in the mirror. The door to the medicine cabinet in my bathroom stayed open. If anyone else noticed my bloated face, they didn't say anything, but I noticed enough for everyone. Frankly, I was relieved to leave the US for a while. In Europe, I was highly unlikely to run into anyone I knew.

During my most anxious times, I obsessed about death. I was stalked by kidney failure. People died from kidney failure. Dr. Kraus thought I had enough kidney function to last until the end of the year. What if he was wrong? What if, what if, what if....

I tried not to let Joe know how ill and scared I felt. I didn't want to ruin our "non-honeymoon" with constant complaints about various ailments and fears. Years later, when we were reminiscing about this time in our marriage, I told Joe how sick I felt during a lot of this trip.

He wasn't pleased with me or himself. "Why would you hide how you were feeling from me? I'm supposed to know these things so I can take care of you."

At the same time, he seemed disgusted with himself. Joe, the Eagle Scout, had pledged long ago to "help other people at all times."

"What's wrong with me?" he asked himself incredulously. "Why didn't I notice how sick you were?"

On September 19, 2004, Joe and I flew out of Dulles Airport in Virginia, to begin our European excursion. This would be the longest trip we'd taken together, and we found that we were good traveling companions. We spent our Paris days strolling hand in hand all over the city, stopping along the Champs Elysée for meals at any sidewalk café that looked appealing, perusing eye-watering boutiques in the quaint back alleys off the main rues, and visiting famous Parisian landmarks such as the Louvre, and the Eiffel Tower. The place I enjoyed vising most in the City of Lights was the Shakespeare and Company bookstore on the Left Bank. While the original store had closed in 1941, walking through this one, where Baldwin, Hughes, and Wright, among so many others had trod and read their work, was beyond surreal.

By the time we arrived in Nice, France's fifth most populous city, I was more than ready for a rest. I'd come to the right place. Life was slow and easy in Nice, and we fit right in. I'd sleep late while Joe took a run on the beach beside the Mediterranean Sea. Then we'd have a leisurely midday meal in the first-floor café of our hotel. My favorite noontime fare was coffee, salad niçoise (sans anchovies), a croissant or baguette and Perrier. Almost every day, I'd ask Joe, "Why do croissant and Perrier taste so much better in France than in the United States?" Everyday Joe would roll his eyes and give me the same answer, "because we're in France, baby!"

Joe and I were having a grand time, but I was beginning to wilt. Boarding the plane to Barcelona, I found myself longing for a pair of ruby slippers so, like Dorothy, I could click my heels three times and be back in Washington, DC. But first to Barcelona. As spent as I felt on some days, I couldn't resist the city's infectious atmosphere. I rallied enough to roam the crowded Ramblas and marvel at the "human statues," and tour the strange, but fascinating "Casa Batllo," a masterpiece by Spanish architect Antoni Gaudi.

On October 6, our last day in the city. Joe and I got up at 3:00 in the morning Barcelona time to watch renown journalist and our friend (the now late) Gwen Ifill moderate the 2004 Vice Presidential debate between John Edwards and Dick Cheney. Maybe getting up in the middle of the night while on vacation to watch a political debate was crazy. But Gwen was the first African American woman to have this prestigious role. I remember that we howled with glee when Gwen had to verbally "check" Cheney a few times when he wanted to talk out of turn. What a treat.

Our brief time in Madrid and London and the travel back home to the United States was a blur. By the time we touched down at National Airport in DC, I had difficulty walking. This meant that water and waste were pooling in my body. I didn't want Joe to see my legs. They looked like I had elephantiasis—not very attractive for a new bride. As much as I hated to think about it, I knew I needed to see a doctor soon.

Dr. Krauss lived up to his word and talked about my case with his colleague, Jack Moore at Washington Hospital Center. Joe and I arrived back in DC on the evening of October 8th. On Wednesday, October 13, I was sitting in an examining room waiting to see Dr. Moore. Joe wanted to come with me to this first visit, but I insisted he go to work. We'd only been married for six months and after twenty years of single life, I sometimes had trouble letting him take care of me.

As I sat waiting for the doctor, I wondered how much Joe would have to take care of me in the future. I could be on dialysis in a few months. I wondered if my responsible, dependable husband had signed up for more than he could handle.

"Ms. Watson?" I looked up to see a stocky, balding, White man in a white coat walk briskly into the examining room.

"Jack Moore," he said formally, sticking a beefy hand out for me to shake.

Krauss had described Moore as a former army doctor. I could see this man giving orders.

Moore looked me straight in the eye when he spoke. "You look good, Ms. Watson, but I've read your chart. You've had a pretty good go with FSGS, and it's not done with you yet."

My breath quickened. I didn't know whether to feel glad that this new doctor understood what I'd been through or scared that he saw trouble in my future.

"Can you help me, doctor?" I asked in as calm a voice as I could manage.

"Well, Ms. Watson," Dr. Moore said folding his arms across his chest. "Let me ask you something. Are you punctual?"

What kind of question is that, I thought. Had this doctor taken one look at me and decided that I ran on CP time? "Yes, I'm punctual," I answered, defensively. "In fact, Doctor, I tend to arrive at appointments early."

"That's good, Ms. Watson," Moore responded, "because I don't have time to wait around for people. Get up on the table please so I can examine you."

The examining table was set higher than I expected and I struggled to maintain my dignity as I climbed onto it.

"Your glands feel normal," he said after feeling my neck. "Your heart sounds good. You have a slight heart murmur, but nothing I'd worry about now. Give me your arm," he said as he unrolled a blood pressure cuff that was hanging on the wall.

"Not bad, Ms. Watson. 135/78." Dr. Moore nodded his head in approval, and I exhaled. I'd been worried about my pressure.

"Now, step on the scale for me."

"Shit," I whispered under my breath. My weight was another number that could send me into a downward spiral.

"Is this your normal weight, Ms. Watson, 136?"

"Give or take a pound or two" I answered with relief. I felt puffy and was sure I'd weigh more.

"Okay, Ms. Watson," Dr. Moore said, turning toward the door. "We're done for now until I can get a look at your labs from today. I want to see you back here in a month." I caught myself before I almost shouted after him. "Dr. Moore, please, just a minute. You didn't answer my question. Can you help me?"

The doctor's whole body seemed to soften a bit as he turned and looked at me. When he spoke to me, his tone was softer too. "Ms. Watson, yes, I can help you," he said, "but I can't do anything to stop your kidneys from failing. Now, the good Lord can do whatever he wants, but from what I can see in your records, Dr. Krauss is right. I'll get some new labs, but you're heading for dialysis in the next few months. I can help you get ready for that, and I'll take care of you while you're in treatment."

Maybe I should have had Joe come with me. I needed him by my side. I felt weak—like I might need help getting down from the examining table. Where is the tough South Philly girl I used to be? I wondered. Then I realized that Dr. Moore was still talking.

"I'm going to see how long we can put off dialysis. We need time to get you in to see Dr. Aquino, the vascular surgeon. He'll evaluate you for a fistula and you can start getting your arm ready. A fistula access will be much safer than the catheter you had in your neck before—much less chance of infection."

As much as I'd wanted more information from Moore, the more he talked, the more nervous I got. I was unprepared for his recitation of what the future had in store for me— dialysis, fistulas, infections. But I tried to control the shiver in my voice. As sympathetic as Moore was at that moment, I didn't want this army doctor to think I was weak.

"Dr. Moore," I said, "I haven't been feeling well. My stomach is always upset, my food doesn't digest well, and I have frequent bouts of diarrhea. Is there anything you can give me or that I can do?"

"Ms. Watson, your transplanted kidney is not doing its job. That's why you're feeling so badly. One of your transplant medications is likely exacerbating the diarrhea but taking you off that medicine now might make things worse. I'd suggest Imodium for diarrhea and Tums for nausea, gas, and bloating. These over-the-counter drugs should make you feel a little more comfortable. Call me if you start feeling worse or if you have trouble breathing. Okay, Ms. Watson?"

I shook my head yes. I couldn't summon the energy to speak.

Moving toward the door, Moore added, "pick up your lab slips from the young lady outside at the desk. She'll point you toward the lab. Also, make an appointment with her for some time in November, and don't be late."

BERNARDINE WATSON

∼

DESPITE MY UNCERTAIN FUTURE, Joe and I tried to enjoy life, adopting a "Ram Dass, be here now" approach to every day. While I never felt fully healthy, being with Joe was a great tonic. My husband worried about me, but never babied me or treated me like an invalid. We went to the movies, to dinner, to live music performances at the Kennedy Center, Bohemian Caverns, and Twins Jazz. We also took long walks around our neighborhood and in nearby Rock Creek Park.

These early months as a married couple weren't always smooth and easy for Joe and me. While we loved each other deeply, we were two fully formed, headstrong, adults in our fifties trying to blend our separate lives into a harmonious whole. Sometimes our fights over money, house renovations, chores, and children were blazing. Sometimes, the stress of my ever-present illness only added fuel to those fires. Fortunately, despite all the issues we faced, Joe and I were also smart and experienced enough to know when to turn down the flame.

Thankfully, my new husband and I also had the benefit of satisfying work. Joe, a diehard journalist, was the editor of *FOCUS*, the magazine published by the Black think tank, Joint Center for Political and Economic Studies. *FOCUS* targeted Black elected officials and covered issues affecting the Black community. I, on the other hand, was fortunate enough to have secured a long-term consulting contract with the William Penn Foundation in Philadelphia, helping to guide their approach to youth programming in under-resourced communities.

My work with William Penn provided intellectual stimulation that felt particularly important now that FSGS had me in its grip. I liked knowing that my brain still worked well, even though my kidneys didn't. Just as important, however, was the independence I derived from my work. When Joe and I married in the spring, our salaries were close to equivalent. Despite my deteriorating health, I worked hard to generate consulting work so I could continue taking care of myself and paying my own way. As far as I was concerned, Joe didn't marry someone he'd have to support financially. On days when I didn't feel well, I often worked anyway.

Sometimes the voice in my head sounded just like my father's. Daddy always pushed us to work hard, whether at schoolwork or housework, sick or well. In fact, he worked himself like a dog. Daddy was tough—often too tough. But on some days, I was glad for the grit he bequeathed to me. I needed every bit of it now.

The William Penn assignment didn't require much travel, but I relished the opportunity to make occasional trips to Philadelphia for meetings. I'd put on my best outfit, my coolest jewelry, the most fashionable, yet comfortable shoes in my closet, and board Amtrak. According to those familiar with my situation, I didn't look sick. So, I was just another businessperson riding the Acela up and down the Northeast Corridor. As folks in my old South Philly neighborhood use to say, "Dark skin hides a multitude of sin." These people were usually talking about how black skin could often hide the effects of the hard living so many Black people in my neighborhood did. In my case, I was happy that my coloring kept the effects of FSGS from showing up too obviously on my face.

Joe accompanied me on my November visit with Dr. Moore. He insisted, and I didn't resist this time. Besides, I wanted my doctors to meet my husband. Throughout my illness, I'd advocated well for myself in the health care system, but as a journalist,

Joe was trained to be skeptical, ask questions, and not back down until he got answers. Also, I was proud to have this confident, intelligent, assertive, Black man by my side.

"Ms. Watson, Mr. Davidson, I'd like you to meet Dr. Alejandro Aquino," Dr. Moore said, as a short, portly, smiling, Asian man walked into the exam room. "Alex, meet Ms. Watson and her husband, Mr. Davidson. Dr. Aquino is one of the top vascular surgeons in the country." Despite Aquino's height, he had a booming voice. He also had an accent. I'd find out later that he is Filipino.

"Hello, Ms. Watson, Mr. Davidson," he said warmly and with an ear-to-ear grin.

Aquino was so different from Dr. Moore, or Dr. Rudnick for that matter, both of whom always seemed so serious and stern.

"I'm glad to meet you, of course," Aquino continued pleasantly putting his arm around my shoulder, "but I'm sorry to see you here in this clinic."

Suddenly he was serious. "How can I help?"

Dr. Moore spoke up before I could answer.

"Ms. Watson is going to start dialysis soon—and she's going to need a fistula. I want you to look at her arm."

Joe and I looked at each other with dismay. We were still getting used to the reality Moore spoke about so easily. I expected Dr. Aquino to ask to see my arm. Instead, he pulled up a chair across from me, sat down, and asked, "Tell me what's going on, Ms. Watson."

Aquino listened, making soft sympathetic murmurings, as I gave him the pertinent facts of my story. I seemed to have his full attention.

"Are you on the transplant list, Ms. Watson?"

I looked at Aquino with surprise. Transplant list? I'd just lost the kidney my sister Alice gave me. Was I eligible for another one? I looked over at Joe and could see that he was listening to Aquino with great interest. Then I turned to look at Dr. Moore.

"Alex, Alex, we haven't gotten that far yet," Dr. Moore interjected. "I'm going to talk with her about transplantation. Now we need to work on getting her a dialysis access."

Dr. Aquino didn't respond to Doctor Moore but directly to me and Joe.

"Yes, Ms. Watson, Mr. Davidson. You must start thinking about another transplant—that's what's best, you know." His face became a mask of seriousness. "You're right-handed, Ms. Watson?"

I slowly nodded yes.

"Let me see your left arm, then. We'll leave the right one alone."

Aquino took my arm as if he were going to kiss my hand and began feeling and turning my forearm gently this way and that. Apparently, this examination was taking too long for Dr. Moore.

"Ms. Watson, I'm going down the hall to see another patient. When you're done with Dr. Aquino, please come down to the desk and ask them to page me. I'd like to see you before you go."

I nodded at Dr. Moore but was more interested in Dr. Aquino's detailed examination of my arm.

"You have very small veins, Ms. Watson," Aquino said patting my arm, "but we can work with that."

Dr. Aquino pulled a pamphlet and ink pin from his pocket and motioned Joe to come closer. He then began to speak very precisely to me and Joe as if he were making sure we could understand him despite his accent.

"To create the AV fistula in your arm, I need to connect an artery to a vein. The artery is the blood vessel that carries blood away from your heart. The vein is the blood vessel that carries blood back toward your heart."

Aquino traced the artery and vein on the pamphlet with his pin, looking up at Joe and me to make sure we were following his explanation.

"Connecting these two vessels makes it easier to place the needles for dialysis and allow your blood to flow out of your body through the dialysis machine for cleaning and back into your body quickly. As I said, Ms. Watson, you have very small veins, so we must start preparing your arm for the fistula surgery. Do you play tennis?" Aquino asked, looking up at me with a sly grin.

What? What? Was this man joking? Why were we talking about tennis? Suddenly Aquino didn't seem so charming.

"No doctor, I don't play tennis," I said, the annoyance coming through in my voice.

"I'm sorry, Ms. Watson," Dr. Aquino said shaking his head. "I guess this is not the time for jokes. I asked because squeezing a tennis ball or any small hard ball can help build up the blood vessels and muscles in your arm, so more blood can be pushed through the fistula during dialysis. I want you to work with the ball for 10 to 20 minutes, several times a day. Can you get hold of a tennis ball, Ms. Watson?"

I stared at the doctor, momentarily unable to answer him. Everything was happening so quickly. Joe could see my distress and jumped with an answer.

"Of course, Dr. Aquino, we can find a tennis ball. If we don't have one at home, they're easy enough to buy."

I looked over at Joe and mouthed "thank you" as he stood to get our coats. But Aquino wasn't quite done with us.

TRANSPLANT: A MEMOIR

"When will you be back to see Dr. Moore, Ms. Watson?" he asked.

Again, Joe spoke up for me.

"I think he wants to see her back in a month."

"That timing is good," Aquino said as he headed for the door. "Make an appointment to see me on that same day. I'll see how your arm is doing. You know, once we do the surgery, the fistula will still have to mature for several weeks. Let's hope you don't need an access for a while."

"I wish I didn't need an access at all," I responded.

Dr. Aquino turned around and looked at me. His face melted with compassion.

"I'm so sorry, Ms. Watson, I know this is tough. FSGS is very bad." Aquino made a face like a child who didn't want to eat her vegetables. "But we will take good care of you." Then Aquino shook his finger at me and Joe and spoke with mock toughness.

"Talk to Dr. Moore about a second transplant. See you next month."

I wanted to scream. My new husband was becoming good at reading the emotions in my face.

"Everything will be okay baby," he said, taking my hand in his. "I'll be here whatever happens. Let's see what Jack Moore has to say."

I followed Joe down the hall, but I only believed part of what he'd said. I knew for certain that he'd be with me no matter what happened. That's the kind of man Joe is. However, at that moment, I didn't believe everything would be okay.

"Ms. Watson, right?" asked the young woman at the desk. "Dr. Moore had another appointment but wants to see you back here in about a month," she said as she searched the calendar for a date. "How's Thursday, December 16?"

Joe and I both shrugged and shook our heads yes simultaneously. What else did I have to do that was more important than saving my own life? I'd take any date she had.

I kept the appointment with Dr. Moore on the morning of December 16th, although I didn't feel well at all. My stomach was upset. I was having trouble digesting food. My feet were swollen, and I was exhausted. Still, hiding how truly bad I felt, I convinced Joe that I could make the twenty-minute drive to Washington Hospital Center by myself. I figured that I might as well get used to driving when I didn't feel well. If I were to believe the doctors, I'd be on dialysis soon. Joe wouldn't be able to drive me all the time.

"I want you to come in on Monday to have a catheter inserted into your chest," Dr. Moore said after examining me. "You'll need dialysis before your arm is ready for a fistula. Someone will call you later today or tomorrow to tell you where to go on Monday. In the meantime rest and go to the emergency room if you have trouble breathing. Okay, Ms. Watson?"

"I'll be okay until Monday, doctor?" I asked. My heart was beating a little faster than usual. I was scared. Maybe I won't make it until Monday.

"You'll be okay, Ms. Watson. I wouldn't send you home otherwise. But listen to me," Dr. Moore said, emphatically, "go to the emergency room if you have trouble breathing and tell them to call me right away."

I took a nap that afternoon and I stayed in bed all day Saturday. My feet hurt so badly I didn't want them to touch the floor. Joe lay in bed beside me reading the newspaper, looking over at me anxiously as I tossed and turned trying to find a comfortable position. "You alright, babe?" I'd nod my head yes even though I wasn't.

"Do you want anything to eat or drink baby?" Joe asked periodically. Can I bring you some ginger ale?"

We'd started keeping ginger ale in the house when I began having so much trouble with my stomach. The soda was a favorite remedy that my mother would give us as children at the first hint of any stomach ailment.

"No, thank you, sweetheart," I whispered. "Maybe later." The truth was, I didn't feel I could digest anything. My stomach was so bloated that I looked at least six months pregnant.

"Should I call Dr. Moore?" Joe asked anxiously.

My head was spinning, and I wanted to try and sleep. Joe meant well, but his constant questioning was making me feel worse. I didn't want to sound cross, so I adjusted my attitude before I answered him.

"No, please, don't call. Dr. Moore will tell me to come to the emergency room and that's the last thing I want. Let me try and get some sleep."

I struggled to turn over onto my right side, my best side for sleeping. Joe sighed and rubbed my back.

Finally, I fell asleep, but after what seemed like only a few minutes, I was startled by a loud pounding noise. What the hell is that, I wondered. I looked over at Joe and saw that he'd fallen asleep, the newspaper askew all over his side of the bed. As I reached over to shake him, I realized that the loud pounding noise I heard was coming from my own body. My heart was pounding as if it were going to jump out of my chest. What is happening to me? When I called out to Joe, I found that I could hardly breathe. I began shaking my husband.

"We have to go to the hospital, Joe," I said haltingly. "My heart is beating like crazy. I'm scared."

After taking one look at me, Joe jumped out of bed and

began pulling on his pants. I struggled to throw on whatever clothes I could find. In five minutes, we were out the door and driving into the night.

Joe later told me that by the time we got to the hospital I was delirious. "You were thrashing around and talking out of your head."

All I remembered was being put on a gurney, rushed into an examining room, and given a shot of something. The last thing I heard was a male voice saying derisively, "her breath smells like a urinal."

When I woke up, daylight was streaming through a window. Joe was sitting in the chair beside my bed.

"Hey, baby," he said. "You're finally awake."

I was groggy but could hear the happiness in his voice. He leaned over to kiss me on the cheek. "I've been waiting for you to wake up."

My head hurt. What in the world happened last night? As I struggled to recall the last 24 hours, I heard Dr. Moore's unmistakable voice in the hallway, and then at the door of my room.

"I see you couldn't wait until Monday, Ms. Watson," Moore said. I couldn't tell if he was joking or annoyed with me. Then I remembered that I was supposed to see Dr. Moore on Monday to have a catheter inserted into my chest.

"What day is today?" I asked.

Joe squeezed my hand. "Today is Sunday, baby. We came in last night, remember?"

Before I could answer Joe, Dr. Moore walked over to my bedside and started speaking to me in a grave tone.

"Your situation is quite serious, Ms. Watson."

Joe's hand tightened around mine. "What's the matter, Dr. Moore?"

I knew my husband by now. He was worried but trying to stay calm.

"Well Mr. Davidson, your wife needs dialysis urgently. I'm glad you brought her in last night. She's very ill. We need an access to start the dialysis, but she has a fever. Dr. Aquino in radiology doesn't want to put a catheter in her chest while her temperature is high. I admit, going ahead with the catheter insertion is risky, but I'd risk it. Without dialysis soon we could have more serious problems on our hands."

I could hear Joe and Dr. Moore talking about me, but couldn't summon the effort to speak up. Perspiration was settling in the folds of my neck.

What's her temperature?" Joe asked, sounding alarmed. "What kind of problems are you talking about?"

"Your wife is in acute renal distress—uremia, sir. Her temperature was 102 last night, but we gave her something to bring it down. Toxins are building up in her system. If she doesn't get dialysis soon, her organs could start to shut down. I can create a temporary, emergency access so we can insert a catheter into her groin and perform the dialysis, but you and your wife must agree to that."

Was I hearing the doctor correctly? A catheter where? Joe began to interrogate Dr. Moore. "Will you do this procedure yourself, Doctor? Is that the only choice you have? What's involved?"

"Yes, Mr. Davidson," Dr. Moore answered patiently. "I'm going to insert the catheter myself, right here in this room. Look, this isn't my first choice. A catheter in the groin is more likely to get infected, but I don't think we can afford to wait. Understand, this catheter will be temporary. We'll take the tube out as soon as possible and have radiology put one in her chest, until we can put the fistula in her arm."

I summoned as much energy as I could to ask Dr. Moore the question looming in my head. "Will I be in any pain doctor?" I didn't want a repeat of the traumatic experience several years ago when that first catheter was forced into my chest at Graduate Hospital in Philadelphia.

"We'll give you something to calm you down and dull the area," said Dr. Moore. "I have to tell you though, Ms. Watson, this will be uncomfortable. You'll feel a lot of pressure."

Joe squeezed my hand again. He looked tired, ashen, and anxious. "I'd like to stay in here with her, Doctor."

Dr. Moore sighed heavily. "I guess that will be alright under the circumstances. Please stay out of the way."

Joe stayed out of the way. He stood at the head of the bed and held my hand, while at the foot of the bed, Dr. Moore pushed a tube into my groin. He was right. The procedure was uncomfortable, even painful, inspite of the drugs he'd given me. I'm sure some of the pain was emotional. The procedure felt even more invasive than I thought it would. Tears began to gather behind my eyelids. This time I let them fall. I squeezed Joe's hand so hard I was sure I'd broken a few fingers.

Chapter Ten:

DEEP IN THE BELLY OF THE BEAST

On Tuesday afternoon before I left Washington Hospital Center (WHC), Dr. Moore handed me a card that read: Fresenius Kidney Care Dupont Circle-11 Dupont Circle.

"This is where you'll continue your dialysis treatment," he said. It's a good place. Be there at 7:30 A. M. Wednesday morning—that's tomorrow. If someone in my family needed dialysis, I'd send them here."

Dr. Moore mentioned my continuing dialysis in a very nonchalant tone. I'd been so out of it after coming into the hospital with kidney failure on Saturday night that I'd sleepwalked through the two dialysis sessions I'd had at WHC Dialysis Center. Now the reality of needing ongoing dialysis was sinking in. But in Dupont Circle? *The* Dupont Circle?

Dupont Circle, located in the Northwest section of DC, is one of the District's most trendy and historic neighborhoods. Home to numerous embassies, think tanks, and other important landmarks, the area is also known for its mansions and other structures built in revivalist architecture.

I'd been familiar with Dupont Circle for years before I married Joe and moved to DC. In the 1970s the neighborhood was known for its bohemian vibe and popularity with the gay community. During those days, when I came to DC to visit my artsy friends, hanging out in Dupont Circle was a must. Also, throughout the 1990s, when Joe and I carried on an on-again-off-again relationship, we would meet at Kramers Bookstore and Cafe in the heart of Dupont Circle when I came from Philly for a visit. Kramers was (and remains) a local institution frequented by all types of DC folks, including neighborhood residents, authors, and politicians. The bookstore had a reputation as a place to meet on a date. Joe and I did our part to contribute to that reputation.

I was surprised that there would be a dialysis center in Dupont Circle. From my understanding, and what I'd seen in Philly and other urban areas, these centers were generally in poor and Black communities. Dupont Circle was hardly poor and had been predominately White for decades. But here I was at Fresenius Kidney Care Dupont Circle, where Joe had dropped me off.

I immediately hated everything about the place, including the guard in the first-floor lobby who hadn't bothered to say hello but assumed, after one look at me, that I was going downstairs to the dialysis center. Once I arrived in the basement of 11 Dupont Circle, at the Center itself, I hated the place even more. The smell, the people— is this what I had to look forward to for who knows how long? Most of all, I hated the hulking dialysis machines. As I looked around the treatment room full of Black people, I thought to myself, *Sure, Dr. Moore. Tell me anything. I don't think I'll find anyone from your family in this place.* The rational part of my brain scoffed at my being so upset. This wasn't my first turn in a dialysis chair.

Not counting the recent treatments I'd had before leaving the hospital, I'd already spent two long months on the dialysis machine at Presbyterian Hospital in Philadelphia before my transplant in 2000. However, those days hardly compared to what I was facing now. Back then, I knew that my time tied to the big, gray, artificial kidney was limited. Then, my big sister Baby Alice was coming to rescue me in a few months. I'd drifted through much of that experience in denial about where I was. This time around, there were no saviors on the horizon.

When I look back on my first day at Fresenius, I see myself as a small, scared, angry girl in a grown woman's body. Overwhelmed by the sights, sounds, and smells in the dialysis room, I steeled my body and composed my face into a rigid mask as I sat bolt upright in my assigned chair. I didn't want the staff and other patients to see me looking as vulnerable as I felt.

Much like the center at Presbyterian, the Fresenius dialysis center was one big, wide-open room where approximately 40-50 dialysis stations—consisting of a machine and a big blue chair—were arranged in rows that formed a circle around a central nurses' station. As I looked furtively around the room, I could see that during my shift, almost all the chairs were filled.

Some of the patients were asleep, while others sat casually talking, eating, and drinking coffee while they waited for the treatment that would keep them alive. While I tried not to stare, I could see wheelchairs, canes, and crutches propped up beside some patients' chairs. How can these people appear so calm and at ease amid all this sickness and devastation? *These are not my people*, I thought.

The room buzzed with the ear-assaulting noise of conversation, carts full of vials, needles, and other tricks of the dialysis trade rolling in the isles, and dialysis machines swishing, beeping, and pumping. Nurses and administrative staff busily made calls and organized paperwork at the front desk. As far as I could see, the Center was spick-and-span and seemed to run like clockwork. Margaret, the head nurse, stood at the front of the room overseeing the entire enterprise, looking ready to set things straight if anyone, staff, or patient, made one false move.

Nurse Margaret had checked me in, taken my weight, and directed me to my station that morning. My chair was first on the front row facing the nurses' station and I had a clear view of the big black and white clock on the wall. Knowing that I would always be able to see the time was the only thing that calmed my nerves.

I'd told Joe that I probably wouldn't be at the Center for long that day.

"I'm probably just here for orientation," I'd told him hopefully. But that was wishful thinking. Nurse Margaret made it clear that I was scheduled for an orientation as well as a treatment.

"I know this is your first day here, Ms. Watson," she said in her clipped Jamaican accent, "but this is a regular dialysis day for you. I'm going to give you an orientation and you're scheduled for treatment too. Your access is working, isn't it, Ms. Watson?"

I nodded my head yes. After Dr. Moore performed emergency dialysis through my groin while I was in the hospital, he sent me to radiology to have a catheter inserted into my chest for future treatments.

"We can't keep going through your groin area," he said.

I surely agreed with Dr. Moore. But having another tube placed in my chest didn't thrill me either. I knew the procedure would remind me of the catheter surgery I'd had in 2000 before my first dialysis treatments in Philadelphia. A radiologist had jammed a tube into my chest so forcefully that I cried on the spot. Fortunately, with this latest insertion, I was well sedated and hardly felt the tube go in. I'd already had two treatments at the hospital using the new catheter, so yes, the device was working.

"Please wait for me at your chair then," Nurse Margaret said authoritatively.

That was thirty minutes ago. Now it was 8:30 and I was still waiting for her to come over. The longer I sat waiting for Nurse Margaret the angrier I got. The room was cold and the harsh overhead, fluorescent lighting in the room hurt my eyes. I pulled the white, thin, gauzy sheet I found in my chair up to my chin to try and warm myself, but the sheet was a poor excuse for a blanket.

"You gonna' have to bring your own blanket if you want to stay warm in this place. That old sheet they give you won't keep you warm."

This advice was coming from the woman sitting to my right who was bundled up in a red flowery quilt. She'd been sound asleep when I sat down.

"My name is Cassandra. This place is cold, and it's gonna' feel even colder once you get on the machine and your blood leaves your body. Girl, I never forget my blanket. You might have to put your coat back on."

I stared at Cassandra, trying to take her measure in a glance. She was a beautiful, round, dark-skinned woman who didn't look like she'd been sick a day in her life. I tried to guess her age and decided that she was a contemporary.

"Hi. Thanks for the tip. I'll remember," I said reaching for my coat. "My name is Dine. Bernardine is my whole name."

Cassandra and I might have had more time to talk that morning, but suddenly, Nurse Margaret appeared in front of my chair. The look on her face made clear that she wanted my full attention.

"Ms. Watson. We give all new patients an orientation so they will understand dialysis and how we operate at Fresenius. We don't have a lot of time today since you're due for a treatment. I'll cover as much as I can. Take these materials home and read these too," she said as if she was a teacher giving me a homework assignment.

Nurse Margaret planted her feet, threw back her shoulders, lifted her head, and started speaking completely from memory.

"Dialysis is a treatment for kidney failure that rids your body of unwanted toxins, waste products, and excess fluids by filtering your blood," she began.

I struggled to keep a straight face and feign interest in Nurse Margaret's words. Even the Jamaican lilt in her voice (a rhythm of speaking I usually loved) couldn't make the ugly process of dialysis sound bearable. I'd almost stopped listening completely when I heard the nurse ask a question that got my attention.

"Are you still urinating, Ms. Watson?"

I glared at Nurse Margaret and sat up straighter in my chair, as a warm flush of anger shot through my body. I hated that she was asking me this information so publicly, although Cassandra had gone back to sleep and no one else around us seemed to be paying attention. It hadn't yet dawned on me that in that big open room, there was no such thing as privacy. At any rate, my glaring didn't seem to have any effect on Margaret. She just stared back at me and waited for my response. After a few seconds of fuming silence, I answered.

"Yes, I still urinate," I said, not knowing whether to feel proud that I could still pee or disgusted that I needed to be concerned about such a basic bodily function. Nurse Margaret, seeming unaware of my dilemma, launched right back into her lecture.

"Ms. Watson, most people who end up on dialysis because of End Stage Renal Disease eventually stop urinating because their kidneys no longer function. You will probably stop urinating eventually, which means your body won't be able to get rid of waste and excess fluids between dialysis treatments and you'll have to reduce your fluid intake. Dialysis treatments only do fifteen percent of the job your kidneys do anyway."

Nurse Margaret paused as if to let that statistic sink in.

I vaguely remembered hearing Dr. Rudnick quote that stat before, but I hadn't paid much attention. For the first time, I understood that as big and bulky as that dialysis machine beside me was, it could only keep me barely alive. Why is this happening to me, I wondered again for the umpteenth time.

I was beginning to feel a little dizzy. Nurse Margaret's spiel was bleak, but it was also just too much. She'd been talking for about fifteen minutes and already I was suffering from information overload. I'd never been good at absorbing a lot of material presented orally. My mind tends to wander after a while. I looked up at the nurse with pleading eyes hoping she'd take the hint and cut her lesson short. But she either didn't recognize the look in my eyes or didn't care.

"Ms. Watson," she said as if she'd never stopped talking, "extra fluid can cause swelling and increase your blood pressure, which makes your heart work harder and puts you at risk of a heart attack. Watch your urine output and let us know if you begin to urinate less frequently. We'll help you determine the amount of fluid you can take in. Once you stop urinating completely, you'll probably have to reduce your daily fluid intake to no more than 4 glasses or 32 ounces—and that includes fluids from fruits and vegetables. That's why we weigh you before every treatment, Ms. Watson, to see how much fluid weight you've gained. You should gain no more than 1-2 kilos which equals 2-4 pounds of fluid weight between treatments. Okay, Ms. Watson?"

I wanted to scream at Nurse Margaret. I wasn't okay. How could she ask me such a question with a straight face? How was drinking only 4 glasses of water a day okay? For all my adult life I'd lived by the "eight glasses of water a day" credo, believing I was maintaining my health and improving my skin from the inside out. Now, water could be my mortal enemy?

The incredulity I felt must have shown in my face and through my eyes. I wasn't sure why, but this time Nurse Margaret responded with a little empathy.

"Ms. Watson," she said, sounding as tired as I felt, "we'll help you with the fluids. There are some tricks you can try to keep yourself from feeling too thirsty—like sucking ice cubes or hard candy. But you're not there yet. We'll help you when the time comes."

Ice cubes and hard candy sounded ridiculous to me, but Nurse Margaret's sympathetic words also made me feel a little better. At least I knew she was human.

"Thank you," I said, as I stole a look at the clock. It was 9:00. Was I ever going to get out of here? "Am I still having a treatment today?"

Nurse Margaret turned to look at the clock and frowned. "Ms. Watson, we're going to have to cut this orientation short so you can get your treatment. Please look over the materials I gave you about the foods you should avoid. We'll talk about that later."

I nodded my head quickly. I knew a little about the dialysis diet from my initial treatments before my first transplant. I just wanted Margaret to stop talking so we could move things along, and I could eventually get home. I closed my eyes, leaned back in my chair, and tried to prepare myself mentally for whatever came next. However, Nurse Margaret did not stop talking.

"Ms. Watson," she said, and then waited for me to open my eyes before she continued. "I think you know this, but I have to re-emphasize it. And that's exactly what Nurse Margaret did—re-emphasized. She raised her voice, which made her accent more pronounced.

"You must keep your dialysis schedule: Monday, Wednesday, and Friday 7:30-10:30. Do not skip treatments. Missing dialysis allows wastes and fluids to build up in the blood, which can not only leave you feeling weak, and tired but can put you at risk of infection, heart attack, even death."

Nurse Margaret looked at me sternly as if to punctuate her message. I nodded, thinking how little she knew about me. She didn't have to worry about me missing treatments. I might be angry and stubborn right now, but I wasn't stupid or careless. I wasn't ready to die or have a heart attack. I'd come close enough to that a few days ago when I suffered kidney failure. I'll be here for my treatments. But don't expect me to like it.

After Nurse Margaret went back to the nurse's station, a slight, young, woman technician rolled her cart up to my chair, adjusting her face mask and pulling on her gloves as she got closer to me. All staff who got up close and personal with patients had to wear masks and gloves—a precaution, I was told, to cut down on the risk of infecting patients.

"My name is Princess," the young woman said. Because of the mask, I couldn't tell if she was smiling. "I'm going to put you on the machine today Ms. Watson," she said, handing me a mask.

Even with a mask over her face, I could tell that she was Filipino because of her almond-shaped eyes, not-quite-white skin, and bone-straight black hair. Many of the technicians and nurses, I saw walking around the Center looked like they were Filipino. My social science background made me curious about the number of Filipinos at Fresenius. For that matter, there seemed to be quite an international crew at the Center including people who I was certain were Ethiopian or Somalian. Of course, there was Nurse Margaret, and I was sure I'd heard a few others with Jamaican accents. How had so many immigrants found their way to Fresenius? Did the Filipinos at Fresenius all know the great Filipino vascular surgeon, Dr. Aquino? Were there any African Americans and plain American White people in this field? I was curious about this issue but not enough to think too long about it. I wanted to get out of there, so I turned my full attention to Princess.

Given her name, I assumed that Princess was pretty. But why saddle a girl with the name Princess? If she'd grown up in my neighborhood, she would have been teased mercilessly for having such a pretentious name, pretty or not. I later learned that the name Princess was common in Filipino culture and in keeping with the group's practice of including honorifics in their children's names. Honestly, though, while I found the young lady's name somewhat amusing, all I wanted at that moment was for "the Princess" to do her job quickly and well. I didn't care if she called herself "Queen."

Princess went about her work, initially taking my temperature and recording my weight.

"Can you unbutton your shirt please," she asked in a matter-of-fact tone as she moved in to wipe the skin around the plastic tube hanging out of my chest with a substance that looked and smelled like the mercurochrome of my childhood. The tube, or catheter, tunneled under my skin and into a large vein inside my body, providing "access" to my blood for dialysis treatments. Instinctively I jumped and winced before she could touch me.

"Did I hurt you?" Princess asked, sounding surprised. She hadn't hurt me. She hadn't even touched me yet.

"No," I said. I took a breath and tried to relax as she applied the cool liquid to my skin. But I was cold, sitting there with my shirt undone. The liquid only made me colder. I watched Princess closely as she cleaned the catheter and my surrounding chest area. I shivered as I sat there with my shirt open. Besides, people were walking by, and I felt like a freak sitting there with the tube hanging out of my chest.

Finally, I felt a familiar, but still surprising flush of saline solution making sure all lines were clear— a feeling that put me on notice that Princess had connected my catheter to the lines leading to the dialysis machine. Momentarily my blood would flow outside my body, into the machine for cleaning, then back into my body again. I exhaled, pulled my coat up around me, and closed my eyes.

"Call me if you need anything," Princess said, smiling with her eyes as she walked away.

∽

I WOKE UP to see that the clock on the wall in front of me read 12:15. I hadn't intended to sleep through the entire three hours but knowing that I'd survived my first treatment at Fresenius, made me almost giddy. After a blood pressure and weight check, I walked out of the dialysis room with my head high. I felt weak, unsteady, and slightly nauseous, but as far as I was concerned, I was doing okay under the circumstances. I can handle this, I thought.

Hurriedly, I slipped into my coat and switched my butt triumphantly out of that suffocating place, onto the elevator, up one floor, and out of the building, not even glancing at the security guard at the desk. I wanted to scream into the cold January air—*let it be known that on this day Dine left the building under her own power.*

I walked up to the Dupont Circle intersection looking around as I waited for the light to change. The streets were full of White people, who looked like professionals or students bustling about their business. The symbolism of White people walking the streets of the Dupont Circle neighborhood upstairs and Black people attached to dialysis machines in a building downstairs didn't escape me. At that moment, however, I tried to push my morning of dialysis to the back of my mind. All I wanted was to get across the street to Starbucks without being killed in the crazy Dupont traffic circle. I intended to sit down and enjoy a cup of coffee. I was certain that I'd be more comfortable in a chair at Starbucks than I was in a dialysis chair.

Once inside, I marched up to the counter and ordered: "a tall black coffee please—no need to leave room for cream." Despite still feeling a little lightheaded from the dialysis, I was happy. My first treatment was done. Now I could relax. I thought I had everything under control. The next thing I knew, someone was holding my arm and helping me up off the floor.

"You okay, Miss?" she asked. "I think you fainted."

What? What happened? I fainted?

I looked around to see a middle-aged White lady holding my arm. She guided me to a table, then brought my coffee over. In a few seconds, I'd composed myself enough to thank her.

"You're very kind," I said quietly, my face still smarting from the shock of hitting the hardwood floor.

"Not a problem," she said politely. "Did your blood sugar drop?"

I shook my head no and thanked the nice White lady again, thinking, I appreciate your help, Miss, but please don't try to diagnose me. I've just had every ounce of my blood removed from my body, run through a machine for cleaning, and then put back in. I don't want to talk about it.

"Well, you take care then," she said walking slowly toward the door, looking back a few times as if she wanted to make sure I was okay. I couldn't offer her any assurances. I just mouthed "thank you," again.

I sat at the table slowly drinking my coffee and considering what had happened. I'd never fainted in my life. I thought only White women in the movies fainted, I half-joked to myself. Once I stopped joking, I began to wonder whether I should go back to the clinic and get checked out. I considered that thought for a minute but decided, no. I didn't call Joe either. I sat in Starbucks until I felt steady enough to drive. I told myself that this dialysis business was ultimately about me alone. I was the one who should decide what I could and couldn't handle. I decided that I would rest when I got home.

Eventually, I made my way back to the counter. The cute kid who took my order remembered me. He must have seen me fall out right in front of him.

"I need to pay for my coffee," I said softly.

"The White lady got it," he whispered. "You okay?"

I looked at the young man, shrugged, and told him the truth. "I don't know."

As the first months of the new year, 2005, galloped along, I hung on for dear life, struggling to accept my new reality. Fortunately, I hadn't fainted again since the day of my first treatment. I also didn't tell anyone at the Center about the incident. I didn't even tell Joe until several days later. He wasn't happy with me.

"You fainted? Why didn't you call me? My office is not that far away. You shouldn't drive right after you faint."

Joe and I had been married for less than a year and I had only seen him visibly upset a handful of times. I could tell by his glare that he was angry. He was right about one thing. Maybe I should have called and let him know what happened, but I wasn't sorry that I'd driven home.

"Baby," I said trying to sound contrite, "I wouldn't have driven home if I was impaired in any way."

Joe's eyes and voice softened a bit as he shook his head. I could tell that he was still frustrated with me.

"You should have at least gone back to Fresenius and gotten checked out. They probably would have called me. Look, Dine, you have got to let me know what's going on."

I shook my head in capitulation, but still felt conflicted inside. Joe was now an editor at *The Washington Post* and had reorganized his schedule to ride into dialysis with me in the mornings. He'd see me into the parking garage next door to the Center, and then go to the YMCA to work out before heading to his office. I was thankful for Joe and glad that he drove into town with me on dialysis days. Having his company on those morning rides made me feel cared for. Some mornings, I needed that feeling badly. But I also didn't want to lose my independence. I'd driven myself home on that first day of dialysis and would continue to drive myself home after treatments. I'd ask for help if I needed it. Joe would have to understand.

I didn't faint again, but on Monday, Wednesday, and Friday mornings, I couldn't shake the feeling that I'd taken a different kind of tumble. I was sure I'd fallen into a surreal, alternative world that couldn't possibly be mine—into "the belly of the beast." What's more, I believed additional calamities lay in wait for me. While I'd rarely prayed throughout my ordeal with kidney disease, from time to time, as I walked to my dialysis chair, I'd whisper, Lord, have mercy on my body and soul.

One of the initial hurdles I faced, besides the dialysis itself, was the food restrictions that people unlucky enough to lose their kidney function have to deal with. I'd learned about the restrictions during my first bout with dialysis back in 2000, but never thought I'd have to endure them again—and especially not for an unknown amount of time.

I'd always thought of myself as a disciplined person who could follow any set of rules if necessary. However, the dialysis diet seemed counterintuitive to me. Foods with significant amounts of sodium, phosphorus, and potassium were big no-nos. The need to reduce sodium in my diet made sense to me. When your kidneys aren't working, sodium can build up in the blood and cause the body to hold on to too much water. This can make the blood pressure too high. I understood that. Except for an occasional splurge on saltine crackers, I'd always tried to limit the amount of sodium I consumed. Who needed high blood pressure or wanted to be bloated with water weight?

But I found it hard to accept that foods such as whole wheat bread, brown rice, beans, spinach, and avocados, were now bad for me. The reasons for these restrictions were laid out clearly in the material Nurse Margaret gave me on my first day at the Center. She'd tried to warn me. These foods, which I thought were healthy, were rich in potassium and phosphorous—minerals that if not eliminated properly can cause severe damage to the heart and bones. Generally, healthy kidneys remove these minerals and other waste from the body, But as I'd been told a few times, "Dialysis only does about fifteen percent of the job that healthy kidneys do."

After reading the materials Nurse Margaret gave me, I resolved to follow the diet as closely as I could. I didn't want to end up causing myself heart or bone problems. I believed in self-preservation and one failed body part was enough for me. But I resented the restrictions, especially of healthy food. Was I supposed to eat white bread now? white rice?—both of which I knew had little nutritional value. I felt deprived and knew more restrictions were coming. Limiting how much I could drink would be next. Nurse Margaret had recently asked me to do a 24-hour urine collection. That meant peeing in a plastic jar for 24 hours and carrying the nasty container back to the Center so a lab could measure my urine content and output. How undignified was that?

Undignified, among other things, is how I felt much of the time during that first year of dialysis at Fresenius—undignified and depressed. Sitting in my chair, I'd look around the room and see people, all Black like me, hooked up to machines and think, this is my life now. Almost immediately, I'd try to talk myself out of this dark thought. I had a life outside those dull gray walls. Of course, thank goodness, I had Joe and my son, Robert, the two people closest to me. And there were others who I knew cared deeply about me—my mom, my siblings, Joe's children, and other family, and friends. I even had interesting consulting work, which I did on days when I didn't have treatment. But when I looked around the dialysis room, I wasn't dreaming. The scene surrounding me was as real as real could be.

One very real part of my dialysis scene was Clint. I'd called him red-eyed Clint from the first day I saw him in the waiting room at Fresenius. My nickname for him came from his blood-red eyes.

To my great distress, my assigned chair was kitty-corner to Clint's. Every Monday, Wednesday, and Friday morning, I had to walk by him, a walk that was only a few feet long but felt like miles.

Clint looked spooky to me. It wasn't just that his eyes were red. I'd dealt with red eyes too when I was on dialysis before. When my doctor told me, they knew of no reason for my red eyes, I did some research and found that dry, red eyes are common for people with kidney disease or who are on dialysis. Due to impaired blinking and tear formation, excess calcium and phosphate can settle in the eyes and cause irritation. But Clint's eyes looked like actual pools of blood. When I combined his eyes with his jet-black skin, which had the texture of leather on the sole of an old shoe, Clint looked like a ghoul. When he opened his mouth, his teeth were discolored and badly broken with some missing altogether. But that didn't keep him from talking. Every morning without fail, red-eyed Clint would find a "special" way to greet me as I walked past him to get to my chair. He usually said some version of the following:

"Good morning, Miss D. You lookin' fine this morning. You don't look like you belong here, that's for sure. No, you don't."

On one hand, I could have taken Clint's comments for what they likely were—a combination of a "kindness," a childish attempt to get my attention, and a plain old "catcall" best not taken seriously. But given my frame of mind on those mornings, I let Clint get under my skin. He represented everything I despised about dialysis. He was an extremely unpleasant, but unavoidable intrusion into my life.

As much as I hated to acknowledge Clint at all, I was too well raised to walk by anyone who'd said hello to me and not respond. Usually, I'd barely look at him as I passed his chair and toss a terse hello in his direction. With all my heart I wished he would shut the hell up and leave me alone. Why was this man talking about my looks anyway? I was at the dialysis center trying to save my life like everyone else.

Some mornings, red-eyed Clint would be asleep when I arrived. If I hurried, I could get to my chair, under my blanket, and pretend to be asleep before he noticed me. Even on those days, however, my reprieve didn't last long. As soon as I closed my eyes, he'd somehow sense that I was in the room.

"Hey, Miss D, you know you sittin' in Mr. Charles seat, right?" Kinda' strange to see you sitting there, but you sure better to look at, though."

Sometimes, Clint would pull "T," who sat next to him, into the conversation.

"Hey, T," Clint would say in his "outside" voice. "Ain't D better to look at than ol' man Charles who use to sit there?"

T was Theodore Wooley, a tall, thin, man whose age I could only guess—was he 40? 45? T had ebony skin and the cheekbones of a Masai warrior. Anyone who took more than a glance at his face could see that, at one time, T was as beautiful as brothers come. These days though, from the neck down, T was a walking wreck. Life had not been kind to Mr. Wooley. On top of kidney failure, he looked and sounded as if he'd suffered several debilitating strokes. From what I could see, his legs were as mangled as crushed soda cans, and when he walked his entire body leaned to the left. The cane he used seemed of little assistance.

I'd overheard more than one conversation between T, his

doctors, and the Center's social worker. He was homeless and had chemical dependency issues. Nevertheless, I'd heard him refuse the social worker's offer to help him find a walker as well as a place to live. Joe used to tell me that he'd see T sitting with other homeless men in Lafayette Park near the *The Washington Post*'s office.

With my eyes still closed I could see T contorting his entire body, saliva running down the side of his chin, as he strained to join Clint in his banter. I knew their whole routine.

One morning, as I lay in my blue chair pretending to be asleep, I heard Clint's unmistakable voice: "Hey, sleepin' beauty," he called to me from across the aisle. "Do you know whose chair you sittin' in? Ol' man Charles sat right there for a long time. You know old Charles died a few months ago," Clint said shaking his head. "He couldn't take this dialysis stuff no more. Wears you out after a while. I been here fourteen years, ain't that right T? I don't know how many more I can do."

T mumbled something affirmative, and I groaned with exasperation. I'd had enough of Clint. Why was he telling me that I was sitting in a dead man's chair? A man worn out by his dialysis treatments, no less.

I knew that nothing I could do would probably stop Clint from blabbing at me. Complaining to management wasn't my style. Besides, I was sure that Nurse Margaret and others at the front desk were already aware of his shenanigans and decided not to bother. As usual, I was going to have to take care of myself. So, on this Monday morning, I turned toward Clint and spoke up, letting my South Philly girl attitude leak into my voice.

"You know, Clint," I said, "why are you talking to me about a dead man? I'm sorry if your friend died, but I didn't know Mr.

Charles. How long do I have to sit here anyway before this is my chair?"

Clint stared at me through his bloody eyes. He seemed momentarily taken aback that I was speaking to him at all. T stared at me too but didn't try to say a word. Unfortunately, the silence only lasted a few seconds before Clint was talking again.

"You right, you right, Miss D. That your chair. Ol' man Charles is gone. People been leaving this place like nobody's business. But you here now and I'm glad to be looking at you instead of that old man."

Clint and T then looked across at each other and burst into laughter, both guffawing like the Gomer Pyle character of that 1960's sitcom. All I could do was shake my head.

I glanced at Cassandra, wondering if she'd been awake and listening to the whole exchange. The smirk on her face told me she had.

"Girl, you can't pay them fools no mind," she said, sucking her teeth and rolling her eyes in annoyance.

∽

WHILE I SOMETIMES THOUGHT Joe was overbearing in looking after me, our relationship was what kept me from spinning entirely out of control during those early days of dialysis. We spent almost all our free time together, like a secret club of two.

Our Monday, Wednesday, and Friday morning rides to the dialysis center were especially important to me. I loved those rides because they felt so normal. For about twenty minutes it was just me and Joe in the car discussing politics like we always had.

We'd leave the house at around 7:00 and while in the car, listen to the political news of the day on NPR's Morning Edition. Both of us were also on the left end of the political spectrum and hated that George Bush and Dick Cheney had won the 2004 presidential race. Driving over to Dupont Circle we'd take turns talking back to the radio, agreeing with reports that Bush had taken the country into an unnecessary war with Iraq.

"Bush is a war criminal," Joe would say emphatically. "Even the CIA couldn't find weapons of mass destruction in Iraq."

"And the stupid country re-elected him anyway," I'd respond in exasperation. "Can you believe that Bush's popular vote total was the highest ever received by a presidential candidate? It might be time for us to look into moving to Canada."

Back and forth we'd go like there was nothing else in the world but us, our left-wing political opinions, and NPR, until we arrived at the garage beside 11 Dupont Circle and were once again face to face with our private war. We'd sit silently in the car for a moment waiting for Herbert, the lot attendant, to come, neither of us saying what we were thinking, like, *Are we really parked in front of a dialysis center? And one of us is going inside?* But that moment would pass, and we'd get out of the car knowing we had to get on with the day. After a brief exchange of kisses, I'd watch Joe walk away from me—out of the garage and on to the YMCA. I'd take a deep breath and head into the Center.

I hated dialysis for the full five years I was on the machine. But after a few months, I began to accept that if I had to be there, I could at least try and make my three hours in the chair a bit more tolerable. For one thing, as Cassandra counseled me, I started bringing a blanket with me to every treatment. I wasn't sure if Cassandra was right that you got colder when your blood was outside the body being cleaned by the machine. But it made sense to me that just sitting in a chair and not moving could make me feel cold in the winter when the heat in the Center was too low, as well as in the summer when the air conditioning was too high. So, my wool red and blue plaid blanket that I'd brought from a Masai woman during a trip to Kenya in 2000, became a constant companion. I hate being cold, so being able to warm myself made a significant difference in how angry I got when I was in the chair.

On some mornings, if I could remember before I ran out of the door, I'd bring earphones and an iPod Rob gave me so I could listen to some of my favorite music during treatment—Miles Davis, Bobby Watson, Cassandra Wilson, David Murray, Wayne Shorter, Bebel Gilberto—anything to soothe my ragged nerves and remind me of my life off the machine. Most days I also brought along a newspaper, book, or magazine, sometimes all three, to help me pass the monotonous hours of blood cleaning. Sitting in the dialysis chair, I was never so thankful that my parents instilled a reading habit into me and my siblings.

My kidney doctors, who made rounds at the Center on Fridays, seemed impressed by my reading habit, always asking "What's that book you're reading today, Ms. Watson?" and reacting with surprise when they hadn't heard of the title. "That sounds interesting," they'd comment. "I haven't heard of that one. I'll have to look for it."

I always wondered if the doctors thought they should have heard of every book in the world, and why they thought we would have the same reading list. Dr. Moore once introduced me to one of his medical fellows by saying, "Ms. Watson reads *The New York Times*."

I shook my head at his statement. Why did he think my reading *The Times* was remarkable? Had he never seen another

Black person or dialysis patient reading *The New York Times*? I don't doubt that I was being somewhat overly sensitive at the time, but I found the comments condescending.

Sometimes I felt lonely or anxious while on the dialysis machine. These feelings usually overcame me around 10:00 when I had about thirty minutes left before the end of my treatment. I'd get antsy and want someone to talk me through that last half hour. I tried not to call Joe or Robert too often since they both had newspaper jobs that came with deadline pressure. I don't remember calling any of my four siblings during that time either. My siblings and I never had much of a telephone relationship. But that's not the main reason I didn't call them. I'm ashamed to admit it now, but back then I didn't want Judy, Linda, or Jerry to view me as weak or needy. My reasons for not reaching out to my older sister Alice, my original kidney donor, were even more twisted. First, the transplant surgery we went through together didn't cause us to stay in touch. Also, I felt guilty about losing my sister's kidney and believed that talking with her would only make me or her feel worse.

After some hesitation, however, I began to call my mother at ten o'clock on most treatment days. At first, I worried that my calls would remind my mom of how sick I was and upset her. My sister Linda told me how hard she had cried when she learned that I'd lost my transplant. But I decided to take a chance. For the first time in more years than I could remember, I needed my mother. Thankfully, Mommy seemed happy that I reached out to her. She never failed to pick up the telephone when I called at 10:00 on the dot. We didn't talk about dialysis, or anything special. However, I believe that hearing my voice was a great comfort to her. I, on the other hand, was surprised at how much I counted on those uninterrupted thirty-minutes with my mom, something I rarely got as a kid when I was only one of the five children she had to look after.

Some days, I didn't talk to my mother because I was sleeping at 10:00. I didn't like sleeping through large portions of my treatment. Frankly, I should be using my time in the dialysis chair more productively, which is why I brought reading material, music, and sometimes even my laptop with me. I watched other patients nodding away and thought derisively that they probably didn't have anything else to do but sleep. I didn't want to appear that way. But there were days when I had no control over my body and couldn't help but fall asleep. Sometimes, like other patients and like me on my first day at the Center, I slept for the entire three hours of my treatment, something common for dialysis patients. I'd find out later that there were good reasons that patients slept during dialysis treatments. Research says that fatigue, resulting from depression, medicinal reactions, anemia, and the general impact of kidney disease on the body, can be a debilitating side effect of dialysis and cause daytime sleepiness. I'm now sure that I had a case of clinical depression.

I felt I had another reason for wanting to stay awake during dialysis—fear. It seemed foolish to me to fall asleep while attached to a dialysis machine. Even though I had no choice, I never felt safe trusting myself to a machine and to staff who had many other people besides me to keep an eye on. One month, I had two experiences that reinforced my fear.

One morning, after sleeping through most of my treatment, I was jolted awake by pain I'd never felt before. It seemed that my legs were being twisted and squeezed like clothes going through an old-timey wringer washing machine. Cold sweat began to run down my back.

"David, David," I cried out for my technician like a helpless baby. David, a good-looking Jamaican, was my favorite technician. We'd become somewhat friendly, talking about current events and my trips to his home island, as he connected me to the dialysis machine. I expected that he'd immediately come running over to help me, but he was with another patient. One of the other technicians calmly walked over to my chair.

"What's the matter, Ms. Watson," he asked somewhat dispassionately, I thought, given the pain I was in.

"My legs," I said haltingly, although my stomach was also now twisted with cramps. I lost my composure entirely and began to sob. "Please. Help me."

"You're cramping Ms. Watson," the tech said in a matter-of-fact tone. "I'm going to stop your treatment. You're almost done anyway."

While the technician fiddled around with the machine, I vomited all over myself. Another technician came over, put cold paper towels on my forehead, and began cleaning me up. In the meantime, my whole body continued to contort.

"Can't you stop this?" I shouted to the techs, tears rolling down my face. I couldn't believe I was supposed to suffer this way. Is this the dialysis treatment where I die?

"Calm down, Ms. Watson," one of the techs said. "Your blood pressure dropped. I'll give you some saline, which should help you feel better."

A cool solution flowed into my bloodstream. I even tasted the salt. But I didn't feel better for several minutes. I reclined in my chair feeling exposed and embarrassed. Sheepishly, I looked around thinking that I'd made a spectacle of myself. However, all the other patients were either watching television, sleeping, or not paying attention to my drama. They'd seen it all before.

I'd seen people get sick on the machine. I just never thought it would happen to me.

Thank goodness both Clint and T were asleep. While I hated their comments about my "good looks" I didn't want them to see me with vomit all over my face. Eventually, David made his way over to my side of the room. As he walked by my chair, he squeezed my ankle and asked, "you alright?"

I nodded "yes," but I was lying.

Before I left the clinic, I asked Nurse Margaret what caused the horrible cramping and nausea I'd experienced.

"Isn't there something you can do to keep this from happening again?" The pleading in my voice surprised me, but my emotions—anger, fear, and disgust were still close to the surface. I listened to Nurse Margaret's methodical explanation.

"This kind of cramping can happen when the dialysis machine removes too much fluid from the patient's body and the blood pressure drops too low."

I stared at the nurse as if she was speaking a foreign language. The tech had already given me this information and I thought the head nurse would know more. I was frustrated as hell. I didn't want to argue with Nurse Margaret, at least not here on her own turf. I also didn't want to cry right in front of her face.

"Why would the machine take off too much fluid?" I asked incredulously. "I was supposed to have two kilos removed. I'm sure that's what David set the machine to take off. I should have been fine, but that was torture, and the saline doesn't help that much."

Nurse Margaret stared at me blankly. I imagined a thought bubble above her head that read "you're getting a dialysis treatment, not a mani-pedi." Instead, she replied pointedly, "Dialysis isn't perfect, Ms. Watson. Sometimes the machine takes off too much fluid. This happens to every patient at some point. I'm sorry."

She may as well have added "and you're not special" to the end of her sentence. I rushed from the Center thinking that Nurse Margaret couldn't possibly be sorrier than I was. I couldn't wait to go home and finish crying in private.

A few weeks later, I was awakened to the sight, feel, and taste of my blood flying everywhere. When I started to scream, technicians and nurses came running from every part of the room. Moving in my sleep, I'd dislodged one of the plastic lines that connected my catheter to the machine, causing my blood to spew in every direction, even into my hair. Some of the staff tried to calm me and wipe up my blood while others rushed to reconnect the tube to the machine. I could tell from the staff's startled looks that the situation was a close call. Who knows what would have happened if I'd lost any more blood? One technician, her voice shaking, admonished me for moving around too much while I slept. I knew I couldn't stop myself from falling asleep, or from moving while I slept. All I could do was hope that sleeping during dialysis wouldn't be the death of me.

∽

By mid-2005, I'd started to pee less. I didn't recognize this change in my urinating habits at first, most likely because I was in denial. Urinating was my one last hope. If I could still pee, maybe I didn't have FSGS. Maybe I wasn't like these other people at the dialysis center after all.

However, when Center technicians noticed that I was coming into dialysis carrying more fluid than usual, I had no choice but to recognize that I was going to the bathroom less and peeing less when I finally felt the urge to go. Reluctantly, I took an honest look into the mirror at my puffy face, a clear sign that I was carrying too much fluid in my body.

Nurse Margaret seemed indifferent to the fact that I was losing an important function—the ability to eliminate fluid waste. She'd probably seen hundreds of patients go through this type of loss. All she said, "Ms. Watson, you should start now reducing your fluid intake to no more than 4 glasses or 32 ounces daily—and that includes fluids from fruits and vegetables. You're coming in too heavy."

I was terrified to lose my ability to pee. The idea of excess urine coursing through my body between dialysis treatments made me feel like a walking garbage bag. Urine was something to be eliminated and flushed. I began to worry about body odor or bad breath. Joe tried to reassure me by making light of the situation.

"As much as I kiss and love on you baby, I'd know if you had bad body odor. I'm telling you, you don't. And even if you did, I'd still love you anyway."

I believed Joe, but I couldn't find any humor in my situation. Not being able to "pass my water," as my Grandma Daisy used to say, was going to be a big insult to a long string of injuries.

I was already struggling with the dialysis diet, trying to keep my phosphorous and potassium levels in check. Now I was going to have to quench my thirst with only four glasses of water a day. I'd never had to limit the amount of water I consumed, but I had to try. Whatever health I had left was at risk. I was scared. I could feel my vaunted discipline and South Philly girl grit running low.

Another side effect of that woeful year, 2005, was my dramatic weight loss, despite the extra fluid weight I sometimes carried. After about six months of treatment, I'd lost almost twenty pounds. I wasn't unique. Many people lose weight on dialysis. When I asked my doctor about the loss, he said "dialysis puts your body in a compromised state, so it's hard to keep weight on. You'll need to eat more calories to maintain a healthy weight."

Frankly, I didn't want to eat more calories, and given my general mood and the dialysis dietary restrictions, I wasn't all that interested in food. The issue was complicated for me. A big part of me loved weighing 116 pounds—lighter than my dream weight of 120. My Black girl thighs and butt were gone, and my cheekbones jutted out of my face like a supermodel's.

Friends told me how great I looked. Joe told me I was beautiful at any weight. The truth was if you didn't look at my eyes, which always had a slightly red tinge, or notice that my face was sometimes a bit puffy, I didn't look sick. Sometimes, being skinny made me giddy with happiness, and I needed something to be happy about. Sometimes, the image of that tiny girl in my mirror scared me and made me wonder if I was wasting away— or wanted to.

In July, a few weeks before my 54th birthday, I realized that 2005 wasn't finished with me yet. I kept an appointment with Dr. Aquino, the charming vascular surgeon I'd met the year before. Aquino tenderly examined my left arm and said earnestly: "Your arm is ready for a fistula, Ms. Watson."

Both Dr. Moore and Dr. Aquino had assured me that a fistula was the safest way to receive dialysis. At this appointment, Aquino told me again how the fistula would be constructed in my arm. "The procedure is outpatient and minimally invasive, Ms. Watson. A fistula also typically lasts longer than a catheter and allows better blood flow during dialysis treatment. All we need to do is create a strong blood vessel in your arm by connecting an artery to a vein. Since the fistula is formed from your native tissue, there will be much less chance of clots or infection."

I trusted Aquino. While I didn't like the idea of more surgery, I wanted the ugly, bothersome catheter out of my chest. I worried constantly about keeping the contraption clean, dry, and out of the way when I was taking a shower, getting dressed, or even making love to my husband. I looked forward to being rid of the unsightly thing.

The problem was, once the surgery was completed, I hated the fistula in my arm as much as I'd hated the catheter in my chest. Two days after the fistula surgery, when I was home alone, I gingerly unwrapped the white gauzy bandages on my arm to find the most hideous scar I'd ever seen. The giant gash ran from just below my shoulder to a little past the bend on the inside of my elbow. There were two huge, hideous lumps at the top of the scar and the entire wound was surrounded by shriveled, discolored skin. While I knew that the incision was fresh and needed to heal, the extensive damage I saw told me that my arm would never look normal. I'd expected discomfort from the fistula surgery, and even some level of scarring, but not disfigurement. According to both Moore and Aquino, I now had the "gold standard of access options." But all I could do when I looked at my arm was cry. Joe wasn't home so I didn't have to worry about upsetting him. I threw myself a tsunami of a pity party, crying for my beautiful, brown left arm and for all the sleeveless summer dresses I swore I'd never wear.

By September, the fistula was healed enough for me to be "on the needle" like most of the other patients on my shift. Being "on the needle" meant having two 15-gauge needles inserted into my fistula, which were then attached to tubes that carried my blood to and from the dialysis machine.

Initially, I was terrified of the needles. I'd never seen needles so big. Among patients, the pain they caused was legendary. At the recommendation of one of the nurses, for about two weeks, I rubbed my arm with Lidocaine cream, a numbing agent, before the needles were inserted. However, I quickly gave up that folly for two reasons. First, the cream didn't do much to reduce the pain of the needles. When I felt the hurt, sting, and burn of the first needle going into my arm, I yelled at David, my favorite technician, thinking he was sticking me too hard.

"Darn, David," I shrieked, catching myself before I screamed out an obscenity. "It's not supposed to hurt that much."

David, another no-nonsense Jamaican like Nurse Margaret, responded, "Look, Ms. Watson. I'm sorry for your pain, but I'm not sticking you hard. No matter what anyone has told you, the needles hurt whether you use Lidocaine or not, especially with a new fistula. You'll just have to get used to them. Would you like someone else to stick you?"

I had the choice of picking another technician but shook my head, no. If I had to take the needle, I'd rather David stick me. Besides, what would be the point of starting over?

The second reason I gave up on the Lidocaine is because of the ribbing I took from Clint and T, and even my row mate Cassandra. They teased me mercilessly for being so scared of pain. I couldn't have that. If they could get used to being stuck, I'd have to learn to bear it also.

2005, my first full year of dialysis, took its toll on my mind and body. I was forced to give up food that was good for me and accept realities like persistent thirst, a mangled arm, and regular, unavoidable, pain. Also, by that fall, I'd stopped urinating altogether.

Throughout that year, I'd continued to work on small consulting projects—primarily reports and interviews for foundation clients. Looking back, I don't know how I managed to carry out the work given my physical and mental state. I believe now that I plowed ahead with the assignments to ensure that my brain and intelligence weren't being "cleansed" away in the dialysis process. I also didn't want to be financially dependent on Joe. However, toward the end of the year, I began to think seriously about giving up consulting. An egregious disease had robbed me of normal life, and shockingly, an essential human function—urination. I was at the mercy of a machine to do my body's work.

I struggled with the decision to stop accepting consulting assignments, scoffing sometimes at the idea of not working. I watched patients who headed to a full day of work after a morning of dialysis treatment or came to dialysis straight from working overnight. Were they any less exhausted than me? I'd also heard that some patients didn't work and received disability benefits because they were on dialysis.

I did my research and learned that being on a consistent dialysis regimen made me eligible for disability payments. Still, I questioned whether I should collect disability funds. Joe was working and would gladly take care of me.

I thought back over the past twenty years of my life and my ongoing struggle, often alone and in secret, to take care of myself. I remembered how I'd insisted on taking off several months in 2000 after my first transplant. That the transplant didn't work as expected was a grave disappointment, but I was sure I benefited, mentally and physically from allowing myself to fully heal after the surgery.

I decided to apply for disability benefits by asking myself a question that has since become a mantra in my life: "If I don't put myself first, who will?" I'd worked hard throughout my adult life and paid into the Social Security fund. Now I was sick and needed to take care of myself. I approached Dr. Veis, a woman nephrologist on Dr. Moore's team, to sign my disability application. I liked and trusted her, and as I suspected she would, she signed the papers without comment or hesitation. Not having to meet client expectations was a welcome relief. But I still had a job to do. I had to save my sanity and my life.

Chapter Eleven:
AN EDUCATION

I'm proud of how hard I worked for my academic education—working sometimes full-time and sometimes part-time while raising my son as a single parent and earning two degrees from Temple University in Philadelphia. When I earned my first degree in 1975, a college education was uncommon in my family—nuclear or extended. However, the years I spent on dialysis at Fresenius Kidney Care Dupont Circle gave me a different kind of schooling once I opened my eyes wide enough to learn something.

By February 2006, about a year after I started dialysis, I shut down the telephone line to my consulting practice and stopped accepting assignments. My business number, where clients could reach me directly by phone or fax, had been a great source of satisfaction. But why did I need a business number now? That life seemed over. The only real business I had now was staying alive.

I let a few important clients know that I was hanging up my shingle and why. Most of these people were colleagues I'd acquired throughout my career and who knew about my first transplant, mainly because I'd had to let them know for professional reasons. They didn't seem surprised by my news. All wished me well. Their reactions made me wonder if the word was already out in my work circles. Maybe, through the grapevine, some of my colleagues already knew that I was sick again. My first reaction was to feel paranoid. But then I realized that I didn't have the energy to worry about who among them knew what. So, I finished my last assignments and pushed my business cards and stationery to a back shelf in my home office.

As I began my second year of dialysis at Fresenius, something inside me began to shift. The tight spool of anger, fear, disappointment, and grief at the center of my being, began to slowly loosen. I suspect that my body could no longer hold all the negativity I'd been carrying around, and my saner inner voice was finally kicking in. When I think about that first year of dialysis now, I wonder if I was going through something close to Kübler-Ross's well-known stages of grief—denial, anger, bargaining, depression, and finally acceptance. Don't get me wrong. After a year of treatment, I wasn't any happier about my FSGS or being on dialysis. But I had to accept that my body was telling me a story, even if I didn't want to hear it. I had a choice—to make peace with my circumstances or self-immolate.

To this day, I can't say exactly when I began the *acceptance* stage of my grief. Let's just say that I was beginning to realize that despite my delusions, I was in the same bloody boat as everyone else on my shift at Fresenius. We were all Black, on dialysis, and a few steps away from death. I'd thrown up all over myself and screamed out in agony from leg cramps just like others. Maybe I had a few more pennies or years of education than most of the other patients, but these *were* my people. One Monday morning in early 2006, I surprised myself by walking into the dialysis center and greeting Clint before he even opened his mouth.

"How are you, Clint? Hi T," I said in as pleasant a voice as I could manage. Both Clint and T stared at me with what looked like disbelief. I'd spoken before they had a chance to say a word. As I continued walking to my chair, of course, Clint began to shout after me, answering my rhetorical question as if I really wanted to know in detail how he was doing. Although I still didn't want to look at Clint too closely, and would never appreciate his manner, I waved and kept moving. Our entire exchange only took a few minutes. I was on my way to my chair with much less angst than if I allowed red-eyed Clint to annoy me so deeply.

Once I realized that Clint was harmless, my relationship with him and T got a little friendlier. On some mornings, after we were settled in our chairs, the three of us would spend a few minutes "shooting the breeze" about sports, old-school music, or something in the news. Neither man could believe I followed sports as closely as I did.

"You don't seem the type to follow sports, D," Clint would say more than once in any sports-related conversation we had. I'd often wonder just what "type" Clint thought I was, but I never asked. I didn't want to hear his answer.

Of the two men, Clint did most of the talking, probably because he liked to "run his mouth." Also, T had quite a bit of trouble getting his words out. One of Clint's favorite subjects was the "old days" before he was sick.

"I was a bad mutha in my day," he'd say. "I use to hang out with Chuck Brown, DC's Go-Go master, drive a white-on-white coupe, and stay out all night. I never went to bed." T would lean forward in his chair and listen with a rapt look on his face, although I was sure he'd heard this story many times.

As annoying as I found Clint, listening to him made me

sad. If he was telling the truth about his past, he'd fallen a long way. From what I could see, there was nothing "bad" about him now, but his health.

T tried to talk his share of "shit" too, but because of his stroke-induced speech impediment, he had a tough time keeping up with Clint. I was partial to T once I let myself get to know him a little. He reminded me of my father's brother, my Uncle Bobby—a beautiful, charming man who like T, had suffered one too many of life's misfortunes. T and I developed a friendly rivalry based on our hometown football teams—his New York Giants, and my Philadelphia Eagles. Every time the two teams played on Sunday, we'd come into the Center on Monday ready to trash talk, although most of the time I could hardly understand what T was saying.

Now that I could walk into the dialysis center without feeling like I was walking the plank, I was a bit more comfortable. I began to pay closer attention to other people in the room, including my row mate, Cassandra.

Cassandra fascinated me. She usually arrived for treatment 10-15 minutes late. Since I was already seated, I'd watch her as she entered the room, bouncing cheerfully and waving as patients called out "Hi, Sandy!" Where does that liveliness come from, I wondered enviously. How could she be so cheery in the face of dialysis, when I could hardly keep myself from crying?

Even though we sat right next to each other, Cassandra and I didn't talk much, except for a few comments here and there. At first, I attributed our lack of conversation to how much we both slept during treatment. However, Cassandra's friendliness with others when awake made me wonder if my initial standoffishness had made her reluctant to get to know me. I didn't want Cassandra to think I was "stuck up," so I looked for opportunities to engage with her.

One Monday morning, she rushed into the Center later than usual. When I asked if she was okay, she said, "Girl, I just drove back up here from North Carolina. I had to go down there this weekend to see about my father. I'm beat, but I had to come in here and get my hook-up."

I stared at Cassandra in amazement. "Couldn't someone else in the family help you with that, especially since you have to be here early for dialysis? Do you have siblings?"

Cassandra looked at me through widened eyes as she hurried out of her coat. "Could somebody else look after Daddy? Yeah. Will somebody else do it, besides me? No."

Over the next few minutes, while she was getting "hooked up," Cassandra told me about her large, extended family of sisters, brothers, children, grandchildren, nieces, and nephews, of which she was the de facto head. I looked at Cassandra with a mixture of admiration and sympathy. I knew other Black women like her who took on numerous family and community obligations, sometimes at the risk of their own health and well-being. I immediately felt protective of Cassandra and silently hoped she would take care of herself.

Besides, Cassandra, Clint, and T, two other patients—Tracey, and Cammie—made indelible impressions on me. Tracey was a disabled girl of indeterminate age. Her chair was to the right of T which put her directly in my line of sight. I'm not even sure of Tracey's disability, but every Monday, Wednesday, and Friday mornings, her mother or father carried her into the dialysis center. The parents, who looked to be somewhere in their forties, always seemed weary, but as committed to their child as I was to mine. Tracy's arms and legs were skin and bone, and I never heard her utter a word. But she would cry from the moment one of her parents placed her in the chair and left to sit in the waiting room. Tracy's cries would turn to screams when the technician came close to insert the needles and connect her to the machine.

While others in the room, including the staff, seemed used to Tracy's cries, her screams tormented me. I couldn't rest until she'd cried herself to sleep. I tried to imagine what it must be like for Tracy to endure what must seem to her like torment, or for her parents to see and hear their child in such distress. Listening to Tracy cry day after day gave me a new appreciation and gratitude for my own health, however compromised.

I'll never forget Cammie either, who started dialysis about six months after I did. She was a healthy, but somber-looking young woman probably no more than twenty-five years old. About two weeks after Cammie's arrival, one of the nursing staff approached my chair, bent down low, and began whispering so that only I could hear her.

"Ms. Watson, we have a new young patient named Cammie who is sitting against the wall on the other side of the room. Do you know who I'm talking about?"

I knew exactly who the nurse was talking about. I didn't turn and look at Cammie, but just nodded my head yes.

"Well, Ms. Watson," the nurse continued, "Cammie is nervous about being on dialysis and is looking for someone to connect with. Would you be willing to do that?"

Without stopping to think or take a breath, I answered, "I'm sorry, I won't be able to do that. I'm just not up to it."

The nurse looked up at me with surprise, as if she had expected a different response, but quickly changed her facial expression. "Okay, Ms. Watson. I understand," she said, and walked away.

At the time, I was still so self-absorbed that I didn't think much of my exchange with the nurse. However, months later, I felt terrible about my refusal to help a young, scared, Black woman. I was especially remorseful when I saw Cammie and Cassandra, a few times after treatment, laughing and talking like old friends. I could only assume that Cassandra had responded positively to the nurse's request to befriend Cammie when I had not. I'd wave whenever Cammie and I made eye contact. She was polite enough, and would wave back, but, I think she knew that I'd refused to help her.

Years later, I related this story to a therapist who said, "Don't blame yourself, Dine. You didn't have anything to give this young lady at the time. You were taking care of yourself and that's okay."

I know the therapist was correct, but to this day, I wish I'd been kinder to Cammie.

～

THE DIALYSIS CENTER was a world unto itself. From what I could see, the patients who were inhabiting that world with me seemed between forty-five and about seventy years old. A few, like Cassandra, looked well and showed no signs of illness. Others showed no visible ailments, but simply looked like walking misery, I could only guess due to years of dialysis, or other harshness in their lives. Some were amputees dependent on crutches or wheelchairs. Many, elderly or not, used canes. Two people on my shift were blind.

Most of the clearly disabled patients traveled to and from dialysis on Metro Access, a DC public, paratransit service. Sometimes on my way out of the Center to the garage, I walked past them waiting for lengthy periods for this service to take them home. As I passed by, my emotions swung wildly between relief and spine-tingling fear—relief that I had a car and was well enough to drive, and fear that given my current trajectory, one day I too would end up broken and dependent.

Joe was indispensable in helping to keep my illness from eclipsing our entire lives. He meant the vows he said at our wedding on April 25, 2004, including the part about "sickness and health." While he never said this to me, he seemed to want to share my burden. Sometimes he'd take a break from work to stop by the dialysis center and check on me. I'd look up from a nap and he'd be standing in the doorway of the Center. I did what I could to keep disappointment about my health from seeping into every aspect of my personality. On dialysis days, I'd come home and sleep in the afternoon so I could be rested and in decent spirits by the time Joe got in. I wanted a marriage, not a pity party.

I believe that facing my illness together cemented Joe's and my relationship. The ever-present necessity of my dialysis treatments was a burden only the two of us shared. Increasingly, I understood that Joe was in pain too. Sometimes, I'd look up to find him watching me with sorrow and fear in his eyes. We tried our best to bind each other's wounds.

In addition to driving to my treatments together every Monday, Wednesday, and Friday morning, Joe and I established a sacred, Friday night ritual that made the week almost bearable. With Joe's work week and my dialysis schedule over until Monday, we turned our bedroom into a sanctuary of candles, incense, and music. We'd share a joint, get very high and make love for hours. Sometimes I worried that the marijuana would show up in my blood work or interfere with my dialysis treatment in some way, but that never happened. What I know for certain is that being able to relax and escape my day-to-day world was critical to my sanity. Just as important, marijuana heightened my sex drive. I often joked that the dialysis machine mistook my libido for waste and removed all sexual desire from my body during treatments. Marijuana brought it back.

Summer is both Joe's and my favorite season. While I don't remember the summer of 2005, my first summer on dialysis, I remember that in 2006, we made a deliberate effort to relax and have at least a few occasions of normal summer fun. I recall that in the evenings and on weekends we took boat rides with friends off the piers in Annapolis and Georgetown. Joe, ever the Eagle Scout, talked me into going camping once in Elk Neck State Park, Maryland. And with his encouragement, I found that I could still walk the mile from our house up to Takoma Park, Maryland, where we'd have dinner at Mark's Kitchen or Middle Eastern Cuisine. On a few Sundays, I even summoned enough culinary and creative energy to prepare brunch for friends. One of the things I remember best is how slim I looked in my summer outfits—arms covered to hide my fistula no matter the temperature. Now that I was in DC, trying to fit in among an entirely new group of people, I resumed my secret keeping. I wanted as few people as possible to know that I was on dialysis.

I longed to lead as normal a life as possible. Dialysis would never be normal, but I worked hard to follow the dietary and fluid restrictions. Most of the time I did okay. I basked in the positive feedback from staff technicians, especially my favorite, David, when I stayed within treatment guidelines. David was easy on the eye and his Jamaican accent, was easy on the ear. He was a welcome distraction in that place.

"Can I get your weight, Ms. Watson?" David would ask solicitously when I came into the dialysis room after weighing myself.

"Fifty-four and one-half kilos," I'd say proudly, having only gained one kilo or 2.2 pounds of fluid in the two days since my last treatment.

"That's wonderful, Ms. Watson," David would say in an exaggerated tone. "You done good."

I tried to keep my potassium and phosphorus levels within normal range by denying myself favorite foods like tomatoes and potatoes. None of this denial and sacrifice was easy. I found the dialysis restrictions punishing, especially when I was trying to live normally or have fun. Sometimes my willpower would simply abandon me, and I'd find myself drinking as much water as I wanted or needed to quench my thirst, or enjoying watermelon, collard greens, or some other delicious food I could no longer resist. I'd conveniently "forget" about the consequences for someone whose body could no longer process food or liquids correctly.

One Monday morning after a weekend of convenient "forgetting." I weighed in at the dialysis center having gained four kilos (almost 9 lbs.) of fluid weight and with a horrifyingly high blood pressure. My transgressions were immediately obvious in my bloated face, red eyes, and swollen belly, ankles, and feet. *You stupid, stupid girl, I lectured myself. Have you forgotten you can't pee? The extra fluid and waste in your body have no place to go.* In addition to a stern "talking to" from David and other clinic staff, my sins also cost me an extra thirty minutes on the dialysis machine to bring my fluid, phosphorous and potassium levels back into line.

Fortunately, I didn't lose my willpower often. I'm a disciplined person, able to restrain myself most of the time, especially when I know my health is at risk. But the constant monitoring of everything I put in my mouth took almost super human effort. I always felt thirsty and deprived, and even dreamed about water.

∼

I DON'T REMEMBER WHEN or how I first learned about Fresenius Patient Travel Services— a free service that helps patients arrange dialysis treatments when they travel. I immediately saw the service as another tool for preserving some of my independence and sanity.

"Why isn't information about travel provided when people start dialysis, along with all the other regulations and dos and don'ts," I asked the clinic social worker, a young White woman who worked at the Center a few days a week.

"Not many people use the service. People here don't travel much," she said with a shrug.

I didn't like the social worker's response. She seemed to assume that "people" at the dialysis center had no interest in traveling. I decided first, to learn how the Fresenius Patient Travel Service worked and second, to use it.

After my investigation, I found that receiving dialysis at a "transient" facility is complicated. First, is the all-important issue of paying for dialysis in another location. Generally, Medicare pays for eighty percent of dialysis treatment for non-low-income patients anywhere in the United States or its territories. This limits most patients to domestic travel. Most "transient" facilities agree to bill the patient's secondary insurance for the remaining twenty percent of treatment costs. If they don't agree to that, the patient must pay the balance in advance and be reimbursed by their secondary insurance carrier. Given the expense of dialysis,

I doubt many people can afford to pay that 20 percent upfront. Medicaid, which covers dialysis costs for low-income patients, will only pay for treatment in the patient's home state, which makes travel options for low-income patients quite limited.

Fortunately, I had Medicare as well as secondary insurance coverage from Joe's job at *The Washington Post*, so paying for dialysis while traveling was not an issue for me. However, negotiating the dialysis travel process was another issue altogether. The Center's social worker informed me that if I intended to travel, I had to inform her of my travel plans at least four weeks in advance. This would give her time to reserve a dialysis slot for me at an available facility and send all the requested medical files. She also told me that I needed to provide the accepting facility with proof of a recent EKG, chest X-Ray, or negative Hepatitis test. If I didn't have recent proof of those tests in my records, I'd need to have the procedures done in time for her to send the results to the "transient" facility before my visit. Between the financial and insurance requirements and the travel system bureaucracy, I could understand why some patients might not consider traveling away from their home facilities. I was not that kind of dialysis patient.

When Joe's Aunt Thelma in Detroit died at eighty-seven on August 21, 2006, I learned that Fresenius Travel Service could move more quickly than the social worker indicated. Aunt Thelma's services were planned for a week after her death, and I was determined to be there to pay my respects. Aunt Thelma was Joe's mother Margaret's sister and best friend. Since Margaret died before I met her, Joe took me to meet Aunt Thelma and get her approval before we married. Thelma liked me and I liked her. Besides, she'd had kidney failure and spent about two years on dialysis before she died. She and I bonded over how much we hated the scars dialysis left on our bodies and spirits. I drove the Fresenius social worker crazy to make sure she got my medical files to the Detroit facility on time. I even managed to get EKG and EX-ray tests completed and the results sent to Detroit before my arrival.

At 10:00 on Monday morning, August 28, I was in the family pew at Detroit's Thompson Funeral Home sitting next to my husband as the minister eulogized Aunt Thelma. A beautiful picture of Aunt Thelma in her thirties, looking like Nancy Wilson, was perched on an easel at the front of the room. Seeing that picture alone was worth any hassle I'd gone through to make the trip.

Being able to travel to another city while on dialysis, even to go to a funeral, made me giddy with excitement. I still had a dialysis schedule to keep while I was traveling but was grateful for the opportunity to choose my whereabouts, even for a few days.

Patients at my home Center in DC thought I was crazy for walking into a strange dialysis center in a strange city and letting a strange technician stick a needle in my arm.

"You don't know them people," said Cassandra, with plenty of attitude. "You don't even know if those places are gonna' be clean."

The fact is the Detroit center where I had dialysis was plenty clean. The place looked and ran much like the DC center I was used to. The staff was kind and competent, the room was cold, and all the patients were Black. I felt a little dizzy after my treatment but didn't have to drive myself home. Joe was sitting outside right on time waiting to pick me up. Maybe I was taking a chance by walking into a strange clinic, but I needed flexibility in my life even if it only meant exchanging a big blue chair in DC for a big blue chair in another city.

I was intoxicated with the idea of travel. Before I returned to DC from Detroit, I was already on the telephone with the social worker with plans for a vacation. When I got back to the Center, she seemed annoyed with me.

"Traveling again so soon, Ms. Watson?" she asked, glaring at me and tossing her long brown hair over one shoulder.

I nodded happily. My trip would certainly mean paperwork for her, but she'd get no sympathy from me. Because of my dialysis schedule, Joe and I had stayed close to home, not counting Aunt Thelma's funeral. We both had a bad case of wanderlust. We wanted to get away again before the weather turned cool. When I told the social worker that she would have to schedule two treatments for me on posh Martha's Vineyard, she seemed shocked.

"I've heard of Martha's Vineyard, but I've never been there," she said, widening her eyes at my plans.

All I could think to do was shrug my shoulders and respond, "Same here."

To me, "the Vineyard" had always seemed like an exclusive party where only certain people who knew the secret password could get in. I definitely did not know the password. Joe had vacationed on the island with his parents when he was a kid and was now taking me to the party. He had a friend who owned a house in the Oak Bluff community on Martha's Vineyard. When Joe and I got married back in 2004, she'd offered us a week at that house as a wedding present. Because of my kidney failure that year and subsequent dialysis schedule, we hadn't taken her up on the offer. Now that I knew how to use the Center's travel service, we were ready to take advantage of this fabulous gift.

While I was fascinated by the glamour of Martha's Vineyard, I was also a little uneasy about visiting. I'd read that most of the

African Americans who summered on the Island, were elites whose families had owned homes there for generations or who had been vacationing on the Vineyard for years. Would I feel like a "country cousin" around these people? And given my insecurities about kidney disease and being on dialysis, would I be able to relax and enjoy myself? Joe, who never seemed uneasy about anything, joked that I could act as "snooty" as anybody. I promised myself that I would try and enjoy this trip. Since starting dialysis, I'd dreamed about having a "normal" life. Maybe there was a chance that I could even have some excitement and adventure.

Of course, my twin nemeses—FSGS and dialysis—found a way to extract an extra pound of flesh from me in exchange for a week of excitement and adventure. Because I would be on vacation from Sunday, September 17th through Sunday the 24th, I'd miss my regular Monday treatment. Therefore, I had to have back-to-back dialysis sessions on Friday and Saturday before I left. Cassandra warned me about the impact of back-to-back sessions on the body.

"Girl, dialysis two days in a row is killer. You gonna' feel like somebody beat you up. I had to go through that a few times when I missed a session to take care of my father in North Carolina. Now I do not miss. I drive like crazy to get back here so I can keep my schedule."

The treatments on Friday and Saturday didn't kill me, but they took their toll. Joe and I left for the Vineyard on Sunday morning at about 9:00. I'd promised to keep my husband company on the long drive and even take over the driving at some point, but to no avail. The six hours of dialysis within two days left me exhausted. I dozed off and on throughout the entire seven hours we were on the road to Woods Hole, Massachusetts where we would catch the ferry to the island. I remember waking up once when Joe stopped the car along the way. Peeping out of the window, I saw a road sign that said Edgewater, but I had no idea where we were.

"Where are we?" I asked groggily.

"We're about halfway there, but I had to stop to go to the bathroom. Do you have to go?"

I'd been half-asleep, but Joe's question made me sit straight up and stare at him.

"No," I answered emphatically. "You know I can't do number one and you should know by now that I don't do number two on the road."

Joe had forgotten that I couldn't pee, and we had a good laugh about it. That moment of levity set the tone for our vacation—relaxed, free, and together.

Martha's Vineyard was the balm both Joe and I needed. The seven days we spent on the island were filled with all the things that make a great getaway for a couple—good rest, good sex, good food, and good sights. Sure, from time to time I'd find myself feeling a bit dislocated. A few times while I was gazing at a beautiful Vineyard vista or walking past a particularly preppy-looking group of people, I'd flashback to the sights and sounds of my DC dialysis center. No two places could be less alike. Fortunately, I was able to reorient myself. I'd be back in DC soon enough.

I was never far away from the reality of dialysis anyway. During our magical week, I spent six hours—three on Tuesday and three on Friday at the twenty-five bed Martha's Vineyard Community Hospital Dialysis Center in Oak Bluffs. With only three stations, the hospital's tiny center was nothing like the fifty-chair room I was used to. But the over-representation of Black people was the same. Two of the Center's three chairs were filled by Black people—me and another woman. The Black population on the Vineyard was under four percent.

As depressing as that observation was, on both Tuesday and Friday, after I did my time, I tried hard to banish most thoughts of dialysis to the back of my mind. I couldn't, however, banish thoughts of my fistula and the ugly scar it made on my left arm. Despite September's Indian summer temperatures, just like at home, I never went outside without long sleeves.

Joe is the more methodical of the two of us and generally makes our travel plans. Together, we agreed to explore as much of the island as possible. However, it was Joe who pulled out his trusty map and outlined the places we should see. During our stay, we managed to visit five of the Vineyard's six towns: Oak Bluffs, Aquinnah, Chilmark, Edgartown, and Vineyard Haven. We could have made it to the sixth—West Tisbury—too if we hadn't spent so much time sitting on Inkwell beach.

Inkwell Beach, also known as The Inkwell, or Oak Bluffs Town Beach, was only three miles from the Oak Bluffs house where Joe and I were staying. At least once a day, going to or from our tours around the island, Joe and I would find a reason to stop at Inkwell for a while. Reading about Martha's Vineyard in preparation for our visit, I learned that the beach had been pejoratively named Inkwell by White Martha's Vineyard residents because it was always filled with Black people. When we visited in 2006, people of all colors, sizes, and ages filled the Inkwell.

Joe and I spent the rest of our time driving all over the Island. We stopped in Aquinnah to see the famous clay cliffs and to have lunch at the Aquinnah Shop Restaurant run by the Wampanoag Indians, the original inhabitants of the Vineyard.

We spent one entire afternoon walking the streets of Edgartown, where the Greek revival and Federal-style homes look like textbook New England. On one evening, we sat on Menemsha beach in the small fishing village of Chilmark, eating fish sandwiches and roasted potatoes, while watching one of the most beautiful sunsets either of us had ever seen. Despite everything I'd been through, I was luckiest woman in the world.

On the Saturday evening, before we left to go home, Joe and I sat on Inkwell Beach reminiscing about our trip and watching the sunset. While I tried to stay focused on the blazing sky, I was already thinking about the day after next when I'd be back in my blue chair, at my dialysis center in DC. The ever-present knot in my stomach began to tighten. Although I'd had two dialysis treatments while on Martha's Vineyard and been careful about my eating and drinking, I knew I hadn't been perfect. I could feel the serenity of our Martha's Vineyard vacation slipping away and my anxiety growing. What would the scale say on Monday? Would I go into dialysis carrying too much fluid? What would my labs look like?

I didn't want to fall back down the rabbit hole of fear and anxiety. The Vineyard vacation had not just been a time of relaxation for me, but a time of reflection and restoration. While I'd enjoyed traveling all over the island with Joe, enjoying the beauty, charm, and history of each community, I'd also been thinking about the future—my and Joe's future. Joe and I hadn't talked about the future much since we got married. With all we'd had to manage—my move to DC, my kidney failure, and then dialysis, we could barely deal with what was right in front of us. However, our time away on the Island had given me a chance to think, and heading home, I wanted to look forward with more calm and clarity.

I looked over at my beautiful husband who seemed transfixed by the sunset. What did the years hold for us, given my illness? Of course, I wanted to have as much happiness, health, and love as we could handle. I knew Joe wanted the same thing. Well, girlie, I said to myself as I draped my arm around my husband, it's not enough to accept that you have FSGS. You're a South Philly girl, remember? A survivor. You're going to have to fight. *Have you forgotten how to fight?*

Chapter Twelve:
TIME TO MAKE A MOVE

On Friday mornings, Dr. Moore made patient rounds at Fresenius Dialysis Center, usually accompanied by one of the fellows he was training in the Nephrology Department. The Friday after I'd returned from my Martha's Vineyard vacation, I waited anxiously for him to stop at my chair.

"Good morning, Ms. Watson. This is Dr. Brandt," Moore said, walking toward my chair and pointing to a young, dark-haired woman in a lab coat following slightly behind him. The young woman smiled and waved eagerly. I responded with a "good morning" meant for them both.

"How are you this morning?" Moore asked as he reached for the stethoscope in his pocket and placed it on my chest. I nodded affirmatively but didn't speak. In the past, Dr. Moore had asked me not to talk when he was listening to my heart and lungs.

"You're not only disturbing me," he'd said emphatically. "But also, I can't hear a thing you say. My ears are plugged."

I liked Dr. Moore. He was straightforward and could be a little stern, but was friendly most of the time, and one of the most respected doctors at Washington Hospital Center. I'd learned not to get in his way or waste his time when he was "doctoring." Once he'd finished listening to my chest and feeling my ankles for fluid retention, Moore flipped through my lab results. I waited for his comments.

"Good," he said. "Congratulations, Ms. Watson. Your labs are excellent. Keep up the good work. Any questions for me?"

What a relief, I thought. I was always anxious about my labs. Also, armed with my "excellent" labs, I felt more confident asking what was on my mind. I got right to my point.

"Dr. Moore, could I be a candidate for a transplant?" Before Moore could answer, I rushed ahead with this reminder. "Remember, this would be my second transplant."

Moore looked at me as if I'd insulted him. "Of course, I remember, Ms. Watson. I know your case very well—you have FSGS, and your first kidney was a perfect match from your sister."

Dr. Moore's response reminded me of one of the reasons I liked and respected him so much. He had what seemed like an encyclopedic memory.

"We were discussing your situation with our nephrology fellows this morning." The dark-haired, studious-looking young woman standing behind Dr. Moore, shook her head in quick agreement but didn't say a word. Moore continued, "Ms. Watson, I'm glad you asked about a transplant. Aside from the FSGS, you're healthy and you certainly take very good care of yourself. You're one of the best dialysis patients I've had. As I'm sure you heard from the surgeons at Penn where you had your first transplant, your sister's kidney should have lasted twenty years. Unfortunately, the FSGS recurred. There's no physical reason you can't have another transplant, Ms. Watson, and I think you're ready. Are you ready, Ms. Watson?"

My heart caught in my throat. I'm not sure what I expected

from Dr. Moore, but I was taken aback by his unequivocal response to my question and the directness of his question to me. *Was I ready?* Now I wanted to make sure we were on the same page.

"Dr. Moore, I was under the impression that I couldn't have another transplant because of the likelihood that my FSGS will recur. I heard that from another doctor."

Moore looked up from the paperwork he was reading, looked directly at me, and said, "Well, Ms. Watson, I don't agree with whoever told you that. I'm your doctor. Do you trust me?"

I'd never been asked that question before by a doctor and I stopped for a moment to think about the answer. I didn't trust all doctors, but I trusted Dr. Moore. He was no-nonsense, but I could feel his respect and care. Moore had probably saved my life that night, almost two years ago, when I came into the emergency room with kidney failure. He'd performed emergency dialysis on me through my groin. If I didn't trust him, it was too late now.

"Yes, I trust you."

"Good," he responded, "because if you don't trust me, we can't work together, can we? Yes, FSGS returns, but I believe you're a good candidate for a second transplant. Do you have any potential donors?"

A sudden jolt hit my stomach that had nothing to do with the dialysis treatment I was having. Dr. Moore's question had transported me back to those days almost a decade ago when I'd had to tell my sibling about my FSGS, and my sister Alice offered up her kidney. Just the idea of going through all that again made me feel nauseous. I knew my sisters Judy and Linda were tested before my last transplant and had the same blood type as me. I assumed my brother also had the same blood type since we had the same parents. But how many kidneys could I take from my family? I didn't want to ask anyone else for an organ.

"Do you have any potential donors, Ms. Watson?" Dr. Moore repeated, bringing me back to our conversation.

"No, I don't have potential donors, doctor. My husband is willing to give me his kidney, but we're not a match. I'm 'O positive' and he's 'A positive.'"

"I know your husband would be your donor if he could be. Having met him, I can tell. Your husband would do anything for you."

I felt a rush of pride that the doctor recognized my husband's love for me. I wondered how much "Black love" he saw in his practice.

"Yes," I responded confidently. "Joe would do anything for me. But he's not my blood type and I don't have other donors. So, what do I do now?"

"Well," Dr. Moore said, "let's get you registered on the transplant lists at as many hospitals as possible. Being on several lists will increase your chances of getting a cadaver kidney. You know the wait for a cadaver organ can be as long as seven to ten years."

Moore paused and looked over his glasses, directly into my eyes. I think he wanted to make sure I heard his last comment. I'd heard him but didn't say a word. Seven to ten years sounded like a jail sentence. It was also about the same length of time as the average life expectancy for someone on dialysis, which was five to ten years. Given these estimates, I could die on dialysis while waiting for a cadaver kidney. When I hadn't spoken after a few seconds, Moore patted my hand quickly and said, "We'll do our best. I'm going to put you in touch with Julie Trollinger, one of the transplant coordinators at the hospital who'll help you with the listings."

When Dr. Moore walked on to continue his rounds, the nephrology fellow, Dr. Brandt, stayed behind. She bent over my chair and whispered, "If I were you, Ms. Watson, in addition to getting on the transplant lists, I'd do everything I could to find a live donor. I understand you may not want to do this, but you should ask all your friends and relatives about donating. Put a sign up on your church bulletin board, and let your co-workers know what's going on with you. Someone out there is a match for you. You never know what can happen." The young doctor turned and hurried to catch up with Dr. Moore.

I mouthed "thank you" to the fellow, although I knew I wasn't ready to take her advice. I had close friends, but no one I would consider asking for a kidney. I didn't go to church, so advertising on the church bulletin board wasn't an option. I didn't have co-workers or clients, and if I did, I wouldn't dare ask them such a thing. And at least right then, I couldn't bear to ask another family member for a kidney. I wondered if I was truly ready to face the transplant "thing" again, or if the resolve I felt sitting on the beach in Martha's Vineyard was fading.

A few weeks after my conversation with Dr. Moore, I bolstered my willpower and met Julie Trollinger at Washington Hospital Center. She was tall and confident, but not cocky. She was kind, but not obsequious, and seemed to know all aspects of the transplant process—personal, medical, and logistical. During our first meeting which took place in her office in the WHC transplant clinic, I calmly filled her in about all my experience with FSGS. However, when she asked me about my desire for a second transplant, I surprised myself by starting to cry. Julie didn't seem surprised at all. She just handed me a tissue and said, "I know all this must be overwhelming."

She was so right. Her kindness and being back in a transplant clinic had brought up a tidal wave of feelings. I was caught in the grip of two familiar emotions—hope and fear. Just being at the transplant clinic with Trollinger made me hopeful that I might get some semblance of my life and health back. But fear was right there too—fear that my hope to regain a normal life would never come to fruition.

I confessed to Julie that deep down, I was somewhat afraid to start the transplant process again. "What if I don't get another kidney? What if a second kidney fails? I don't want my illness to ruin my marriage or my whole life for that matter."

She nodded as she listened. Her warmth and sympathy felt genuine. Julie came from behind her desk and hugged me. "I see a lot of patients here, Ms. Watson, and I see a lot of pain. I know we're just meeting, but I can tell that you're not the type to give up or let fear stop you. We need to get to work, okay?" I nodded. Julie was right.

I completed the paperwork for registration at the transplant centers of three hospitals—Washington Hospital Center, where I was receiving all my health care, University of Pennsylvania Hospital, where I'd had my first transplant, and Johns Hopkins Hospital in Baltimore. Dr. Moore had suggested Hopkins.

"Johns Hopkins is close by and it's where some of the most advanced transplant research is taking place. You want to be registered there."

Being on these transplant lists didn't bring much immediate relief. The fact that I could wait seven to ten years for a cadaver kidney and possibly die while waiting, made the idea of getting a kidney from one of the transplant lists seem remote. Sometimes, I forgot I was even on the lists until once a month a dialysis technician at the Center collected several tubes of blood from the dialysis machine during my treatment and sent them off to the three hospitals. My blood and tissue information would be matched against the cadaver kidneys that became available. If there was a blood and tissue match between me and a potential donor as well as a fit with other requirements, (size of organ, my accumulated time on the list, the distance between me and the donor) I could be a candidate for that kidney.

What a gruesome business, waiting for someone to die so I could live. I tried not to think about it. Every doctor I'd ever spoken with emphasized that I'd be better off with a living donor anyway—and I believed them, even if that's not how things worked out with my sister. But I had no living donors and could not bear to think about who in my life might have "potential."

∼

"YOU GOIN' for a transplant?" Cassandra asked me one morning, as the technician collected blood from my machine. I wondered when she or one of my other close-by neighbors like Clint or T would say something. Collecting blood in test tubes wasn't exactly a discreet activity, especially when the collection was carried out on the first row of the Center where I sat, for everyone to see. As far as I could tell, I was the only patient on my shift sending off blood samples to the transplant lists.

"I'm at least getting on the lists for a few places. This would be my second transplant."

Cassandra shook her head and rolled her eyes as if she would never understand why I would even consider one transplant much less two. "Girl, they put a kidney in me about three years ago that went bad almost immediately. That thing had to come out right away. I almost died. Now, these doctors can't tell me nothing. No more transplants for me. This is the way my life is, and I accept it. God knows what he's doin'."

I had no idea what Cassandra had been through and didn't think it was polite to probe any further. I understood her feelings. I still had moments of hesitancy whenever I thought about going through all the physical and emotional upheaval involved with another transplant. But I didn't understand how Cassandra could think that this horrible disease was God's doing, or how she could condemn herself to a life tied to a machine. All I could do was try not to judge her. She seemed to have an unshakeable faith that she would be all right on dialysis, something I didn't have.

One morning, shortly after my conversation with Cassandra, I sat down in the waiting area next to Clint and T as we all waited for the Center doors to open. Clint's appearance, especially his blood-red eyes, still bothered me, but like lots of other things in my life, I'd learned not to let it freak me out too much. Besides, I'd sat down next to those two for a reason.

"Good morning, gentleman," I said in an exaggerated tone.

Both men started to laugh, as they always did when I spoke to them this way. I had the sense that neither saw himself as a gentleman and took my greeting as a joke. But that morning, I wasn't joking.

"Clint, T," I said, getting right down to business, "Would you get a transplant?"

At first, Clint looked puzzled, while T immediately began to shake his head no.

"Why you talkin' 'bout transplants this early in the morning D?" Clint asked. "You goin' for one?"

"I'm thinking about it. It would be my second."

"Naw, D," Clint said emphatically, while T just kept shaking his head no. "I don't know nothin' about no transplant, and I don't want to know. I don't want nobody cutting on me for no reason."

Now T began nodding his head yes, in vigorous agreement with Clint, who continued talking.

"I don't trust these doctors, man. The only reason I come in here is I start feelin' sick if I don't." Clint made a face to show how bad he felt if he missed a treatment.

"Another thing," Clint continued, "as long as I'm on this machine, I'm disabled. I don't have to work, and I get my check," he said, widening his red eyes at me to underline his point. "Do you know that three years after a transplant they make you go back to work? I can't work," he said pointedly. "I should get something for fourteen years on this damn machine, right?"

I was sure Clint's question was rhetorical and he wasn't expecting me to answer. But I shook my head yes, anyway, as did T, who hadn't uttered a word through the whole conversation. He didn't have to. He'd made himself clear.

I found the transplant discussion with Clint so disturbing that I turned my body around in my chair so he couldn't see the agitation on my face. I could understand his distrust of doctors. But I had no idea about the choice he'd made. Clint had decided to stay on dialysis and continue receiving a disability check rather than try for a transplant because it could mean going to work. It seemed that people like Clint (and T for that matter) were in a no-win situation. Long-term dialysis would likely shorten their lives. At the same time, having a transplant could mean losing disability benefits. Neither Clint nor T seemed like they'd have much success in the job market.

As I sat in my chair pondering my conversation with Clint, I felt a wave of gratitude. Yes, I was in trouble, but I also had options, like the support of a loving husband, no matter what happened. I didn't know what else was going on in Clint's life, but I guessed that I was in way better shape than him.

Unexpectedly, I heard an unfamiliar but nearby voice call my name. Another patient, Gerald, who was sitting a few seats on the other side of T, was trying to catch my attention. Gerald was a heavy-set, studious-looking man who wore thick-lensed, black-framed glasses. We rarely spoke since he was always busy at his laptop, both in the waiting area and during treatments. He'd overheard my conversation with Clint and had something to add.

"Dearie," he began, pointing directly at me, "I heard you all talking and wanted to add my two cents. I decided a long time ago that a transplant was not for me. I've been on dialysis for about a decade and I'm doing fine. I can sit in here and do my work. I know this," he said, as he pointed towards the dialysis machines. "What I've heard about a transplant is not good," he said emphasizing the word "not" with a shake of his head. "I don't want nobody else's organs in my body. What about you," he asked looking at me pointedly.

"I'm looking into it," I said, telling him the truth at that moment.

"Do what you gotta' do sister," Gerald said. Before I could respond, he'd gone back to his computer screen.

That morning, I drifted off to sleep in my dialysis chair with Gerald's words in my head.

"Do what you gotta' do." Those words made sense to me.

I don't know how much time had passed when I was startled awake by a commotion at the end of my row. I sat up to see emergency medical technicians loading someone, draped from head to toe, onto a gurney.

"What's going on?" I asked Cassandra, anxiously.

The look on Cassandra's face told me that something terrible had happened.

"Girl," she whispered, "Michelle's dead."

I stared at Cassandra, blankly. I didn't know Michelle, at least not by name.

"You know, Michelle," Cassandra hissed. "I think she's some type of albino."

Now I remembered. Michelle was hard to miss. She was a Black woman with pink skin and blond hair. I'd seen her walk in that morning. Now she was dead?

The room was strangely quiet, except for muffled talking between Center staff and EMTs, and the constant hum of the dialysis machines. Patients sat tight-lipped. Even most of the television sets had been turned down.

"What happened?" I asked, incredulously.

"Girl, I don't know. I was sitting here watching TV when the EMTs rushed in. I didn't see everything, but I saw them pump her chest for a while, then stop. Next thing I know they were loading her onto the cart. Maybe she had a stroke. This ain't the first time I seen them wheel a body outta here. Lord have mercy."

As the EMTs rolled Michelle's body out of the room, the white sheet covering her body fell off to the side exposing one of her pink breasts. I couldn't help but gasp at the indignity of it all. Cassandra seemed surprised at my response and reached over and touched my hand.

"Ain't nothing you can do, hon. There before the grace of God go any one of us. You stay around here long enough, and you'll see death again."

I knew Cassandra was right. I did not doubt that someone else would die in that room. All of us were just a stroke, heart attack, or blood clot away from death. I was already doing the best I could to save my life. What else could I do? Sometimes I felt like I was walking a tightrope, trying not to lose my head as that Grandmaster Flash song "The Message" said.

"You can't lose your head," I told myself. *Dig deep and hold on.*

Nevertheless, after I saw the EMTs take Michelle's dead body out on a stretcher, I lost my cool for a while. Every day, when I came into the Center, I wanted to scream. I couldn't help wondering why everyone in the goddamn place wasn't screaming at the top of their lungs. I looked around at the people on my shift, watching as patients laughed, and talked together, slept, or stared at program after program on television. Maybe, the purpose of the televisions attached to every chair was to keep everybody anesthetized.

One day shortly after Michelle died, I admitted to myself with certainty that I didn't want to spend one more day on dialysis than I had to. All the ambivalence about having a second transplant disappeared—even if it meant accepting a cadaver kidney. There, I'd said it. I wanted out.

Regardless of my decision, I couldn't forget the other patients' attitudes about kidney transplants. The choices Clint, Cassandra, and Gerald had made, and the consequences of those choices, troubled me. Why would people rather be tied indefinitely to a time-consuming, precarious routine like dialysis than undergo a surgery that's proven to greatly increase longevity and quality of life? I already knew at least part of the answer to that question. All three of my fellow patients told me about their distrust of the medical system. Their opinions were based on their own experiences as well as the health system's history of racism against African Americans. Almost everyone in the Black community is familiar with the insidious Tuskegee Experiment where impoverished African American men with syphilis were, unbeknownst to them, left untreated so that the United States Public Health Service could observe the natural course of the disease. But was that long ago event the only reason for my fellow patients' attitudes and choices?

Having worked in the social policy research field for much of my career, I took a cursory look at information about race and kidney transplants. An article, in the February 2005 *Journal of the National Medical Association (NMA)*, titled "Racial and Ethnic Disparities in Renal Transplantation" provided eye-opening information. The article's author, Joanne M. Churak, states that while in 2000, Blacks made up 32 % of people with kidney failure in the United States, they received less than one-quarter of the 15,000 kidney transplants done in 2002. Whites received well over half of the transplants completed that year.

Churak also lists six inter-related factors that could be responsible for these disparities: 1) racism—caregivers use racial prejudice to deny Black patients treatment or information about transplantation; 2) socioeconomic status—patients listed for transplantation were better educated, more likely to be White, employed full time and have health insurance than those who were not listed; 3) geographic factors—Black patients were more likely to live in poor areas with substandard medical care with little information about transplant services; 4) reliable, cost-effective transportation—lack of access to care can negatively impact transplant patients' access to quality health care providers; 5) social networks—Blacks tend to rely more than Whites on immediate family, community and church networks which may have less reliable information about transplantation; and 6) biological factors and organ donation —biological differences between Blacks and Whites and transplant matching requirements do not favor interracial transplantation. Since the majority of donated kidneys are from Whites, Blacks seeking a kidney transplant are at a significant disadvantage.

While I'd spoken to only three of my fellow patients and certainly didn't know for sure if more Black patients at the Fresenius Center were pursuing kidney transplants, the issues raised in the NMA journal article rang true to me. I'd grown up in a poor, Black community where racism, poverty, lack of transportation, and limited social networks affected all aspects of life, including health care. When I was growing up, I clearly remember my parents complaining that the medical care at Philadelphia General, which was close to our neighborhood and known as "the poor people's" hospital, was inferior to treatment for White people at hospitals in more affluent parts of the city. I believe that if I'd talked with every Black patient in the dialysis center, I'd have heard many similar stories.

The NMA article left me in an emotional quandary. I was grateful that I had the resources to pursue a transplant. But what about other Black people whose health and lives were being compromised by race and class inequities? Could I do anything about that? I already knew that the answer was no, at least for the time being. I already had too much on my plate. But I promised myself that one day, I'd look more deeply into the issue and do what I could.

Deciding to pursue a second transplant, however, did nothing to relieve the day-to-day trauma of living with a kidney disease like FSGS or keeping a three-day-a-week dialysis schedule. As 2006 waned, I tried my best to hold mind, body, and spirit together. I had no way of knowing how long I'd be on the transplant list or if by some miracle, I'd get a live donor. On some days I lived in a kind of purgatory—between the promise of a new kidney, and the hopelessness of dialysis.

Sometimes, even when I tried to keep a positive outlook, my current circumstances got the better of me. Drinking too much was a constant challenge—not alcohol, which would have at least provided some deliverance from reality—but water. I struggled to stick to the 32 ounces dictated by the dialysis diet. I thought the restriction would become easier over time as I got used to consuming less fluid. But at times, the opposite was true. How, I asked myself, can I deny myself water when the body is made up of sixty percent water? As the saying goes—water is life! Sometimes, not just my mouth or lips, but my entire body seemed parched. Sometimes I felt like I could drink a river. Occasionally, I did drink a river—well not a literal river, but I drank way more than I should have. Afterward, I'd find myself as bloated as a fat tick and sheepishly facing the scale—three to four kilos over my dry weight instead of my usual one to two.

Facing the dialysis machine itself after drinking too much fluid was even worse. Periodically, I had to spend extra time in the chair as the soulless machine tried mightily to remove the extra fluid from my blood. There were times when the machine removed too much fluid from my body, and as I found out the hard way, would send my blood pressure plunging. If I were fortunate that day, I'd walk away with a few leg cramps. But most of the time, a blood pressure drop, for me or any other unlucky patient, meant a fit of involuntary spasms, screaming, crying, vomiting—and a vow never to drink that much fluid again. Of course, I would keep that vow until the next time I fell off the "water" wagon.

Inevitably, my kidney disease began to have a greater impact on my body. Because my damaged kidneys couldn't remove excess phosphorus, my lab reports began to show dangerous levels of the mineral in my blood. I knew from Nurse Margaret's lectures during my early days at the Center, that high phosphorus levels could cause body changes that weakened bones. When my efforts to further eliminate high phosphorus foods from my diet didn't work well enough, my doctor prescribed yet another medicine, Phoslo, which helped absorb the phosphorus but made me constipated…and ironically, thirsty.

∼

ACCORDING TO THE NOTES in my journal from 2006, the Christmas holidays were special that year. I'm not sure what put me in such a positive mood—maybe the idea of a transplant in my future—but apparently, I hung a beautiful wreath on the front door and decorated the house with poinsettia and candles. On Christmas Day, Monday, the Watson-Davidson clan—Joe, me, Hakimu, Jasiri, and Rob—sat around a beautifully set dining room table and enjoyed a delicious meal that I prepared. I wrote that the day, with all of our family gathered around the table, was, "a dream come true," and noted that my son, Rob, kept hugging me as if to make sure I was real.

After a dialysis session on that Tuesday morning, to make up for having Christmas day "off," I took the train to Philadelphia to spend a few days with my mother. Since moving to DC and starting dialysis, I hadn't seen my mother or siblings much. Over the years, I'd been known to be out of touch with my family for extended periods, but now, my dialysis schedule provided the perfect excuse for my absence. I stayed away now for fear that those who knew me best would see what I saw whenever I looked in the mirror: my frail frame; dull, lifeless skin; red eyes; and worst of all, the grotesque bulging fistula on my arm. I was afraid they'd worry—or even worse—feel sorry for me. I couldn't have that.

The visit with my mother was wonderful, scary, and revealing. Mommy fussed over me without too much fretting, only asking once how I was feeling. I also saw my sister Linda on this visit. She and her husband had moved in with my mother since Daddy died. Thankfully, Linda didn't make a big deal about my appearance. Linda and I rarely opened up to each other emotionally, but she gave me a long, loving look and an even longer hug.

I'd missed my mother more than I realized. We still had our telephone conversations at the end of my dialysis treatments, but I hadn't seen Mommy in longer than I wanted to think about. I found myself following her with my eyes whenever we were in the same room and searching her face whenever we sat across from each other. Mommy had turned seventy-eight in May of that year. I could see that her arthritis was getting worse, and she was having trouble walking and standing up straight. When I looked at her face closely, I could also see how much I favored her. For the first time, I saw my face clearly in my mother's face. Mommy was twenty-four years older than me, but the way things were going, I could die before she did. I wanted to live.

A few days before the new year, I sat at the big old wooden desk that I'd brought with me from Philadelphia, and with Joe's encouragement, wrote a letter to my siblings, Judy, Linda, and Jerry, as well as a few other relatives who were of age and I felt close enough to. I asked them all to consider being tested as potential kidney donors for me. Of course, I didn't ask my big sister, Baby Alice. She'd donated a kidney for my first transplant back in 2000. And I didn't ask my son, Robert. I was insanely afraid that, if he donated a kidney to me, one day he might develop an illness that would affect his one remaining kidney. I'd find out later that Rob had himself tested without my knowledge and wasn't my blood type.

I explained in my letter that a kidney transplant would very likely increase my longevity and quality of life; that I was on the transplant waiting list at three hospitals but might have to wait for almost a decade for a kidney from a cadaver; that a kidney from a living donor was a better option, but a kidney from a living related donor was even better. I emphasized that after recovering from surgery, most donors went on to live happy, healthy, active lives and that in fact, our sister Baby Alice was a good example. I hesitated for a moment, still unsure that writing this letter was the right thing to do, and then pushed send.

I often thought about Dr. Brandt, the young intern who'd encouraged me to do everything I could to find a living donor, including writing the "ask" I'd sent to my family. She'd moved on to a permanent post at another hospital and I never got a chance to let her know I'd eventually taken her advice. Brandt's very last words to me were "you never know what can happen." I'd find out just how prophetic her words were.

January 2007 started the same way for me as the past two Januarys. I was still going to dialysis three days a week and struggling to deal with all the complications that came with that reality. Increasingly, I reminded myself to try and find pleasure in the small things—such as riding into the Center with Joe every morning. Those drives remained the best part of my dialysis day.

Around 11:30 a.m. on a dialysis day in early January, I arrived at my front door to hear the telephone ringing. Usually, on a Monday, Wednesday, or Friday after treatment, if I walked into the house to a ringing phone, I let it ring. What's so important, I'd think to myself. Let them leave a message. Besides, I knew the caller probably wasn't Joe since he wouldn't call me at the time. Joe knew that once I was inside the house after dialysis, I rarely let anything keep me from my bed and my beloved afternoon nap. For me, those respites were hardly an indulgence but a necessity, a time of recuperation. For reasons I still don't know, on this day, I rushed into my kitchen and answered the phone.

I still remember noticing how out of breath I sounded, evidence that dialysis sapped my energy.

"Good morning."

"Is this Dine Watson?"

I didn't recognize the voice at all. Who was this female with a British accent? Suddenly, I knew I'd made a mistake in answering the phone. I didn't want to talk to a stranger. But just as quickly, I changed my attitude. Maybe this call was about a transplant.

"Yes, this is Dine."

"Hi, Dine. How are you? This is Julia Dutton at the Stoneleigh Foundation. A mutual friend, Kelly Woodland, gave me your name.

Finally, a name I recognized. Kelly had hired me to consult on his youth development work at the William Penn Foundation. Still, I didn't know Julia Dutton or Stoneleigh. She wasted no time filling me in.

"Dine, I'm the Executive Director for the Stoneleigh Foundation, a new nonprofit funded by William Penn Foundation. I'm looking for someone to consult with me on developing foundational documents for the organization—a concept paper outlining our purpose and to help me think through some initial strategy. Kelly recommends you highly. Are you interested in talking?"

Initially, I found it hard to process what Julia was saying.

Did she mean to call me—the Dine Watson who had just come in from a three-hour dialysis session; who had been on her way up to bed to sleep away the afternoon; who'd hung up her professional shingle just a year ago so she could focus solely on her health? I still remembered some of my professionalism and had learned a long time ago to never turn down an opportunity without hearing it first, even if I felt certain I wasn't interested.

"Yes, Julia, I'd like to talk. I'll have to thank Kelly for recommending me."

Julia went on to tell me that Stoneleigh was a new foundation established by philanthropists John and Chara Haas in 2006 to improve systems that work with vulnerable youth, such as juvenile justice, health, education, and child welfare.

"The strategy for our work," she said, sounding to my ears like the Queen of England, "is to award fellowships to exceptional professionals who will work as change agents both in and alongside these systems. I know you were an executive vice president at Public/Private Ventures and led their youth development work. I'd like to bring someone on board quickly. Are you interested in coming up to Philadelphia to meet and talk with me?"

My mind raced. How could I possibly take a consulting assignment? Was I interested in working? Did I have the energy for it? I was on dialysis and on three transplant waiting lists. What if one of my siblings or relatives responded positively to my letter? I had no idea what might happen in my life in the next few months, the next week, or the next day for that matter. I gathered my thoughts and steadied my voice.

"Yes, I'm interested in talking more, although I'd like to take a few days to think and talk with my husband. Can I get back to you?"

TRANSPLANT: A MEMOIR

"Yes, of course," Julia said, "but let's talk in the next few days, okay?"

Joe was ecstatic about Julia's call.

"Pick up the phone and tell her yes," he urged. "You'll be great at this work." Joe has always been my biggest cheerleader and is sometimes more confident in my ability than I am. He put his arm around me and continued, "you need something substantial to do. I know you want to take care of yourself, but you can handle whatever she needs. Just tell her what's going on with you. I'll bet she'll understand."

I, on the other hand, wasn't so sure. A little over a year ago, I'd stopped taking consulting assignments, convinced that I was "disabled." How could I now take on a major assignment? Besides, my professional skills were probably rusty. I hadn't thought seriously about anything but blood, needles, fluids, potassium, and phosphorous for months. More than anything I worried about having to tell her that I was on dialysis and on transplant waiting lists. I rarely told anyone my health business. Would she still want to work with me? Still, the lure of putting on real clothes and taking the Acela up to Philadelphia was now in my head.

In a few days, I decided that I should at least talk with the woman. Joe might be right. I needed to get my brain working again. No one in the family had yet responded to my letter and who knew when or if I'd ever hear from one of the waiting lists. Maybe I was wasting my precious time with all this waiting. I made a reservation to take a train ride up to Philadelphia.

∽

JULIA AND I GOT ALONG WELL from the start. While she was White and originally from Britain and I was African American, we were of the same generation and found we had many of the same contacts in the Philadelphia social policy world. We also shared enough of the same political perspective, although she was backing Hillary Clinton for president in 2008 and I was pinning my hopes on the young, exciting junior senator from Illinois, Barack Obama.

As we sat talking in Julia's office on an afternoon in February 2007, I was increasingly convinced that I wanted to work with her. I liked her quiet competence. While she was self-assured, she didn't have any of that "head of the foundation" arrogance I'd seen in many other foundation executives. Even her office was modest. She seemed eager to work with me, too.

"Your writing skills and background on youth issues are exactly what the Foundation needs to help us get off the ground. Are you interested?" she asked leaning forward in her chair.

I opened my mouth and said earnestly, "Yes, I'm very interested. I'd love to work with you." At the same time, another voice was shouting inside my head: What about your dialysis schedule? What if you're called for a transplant? Don't you need to come clean with this woman? While I was having this argument inside my head, Julia kept talking.

"Great! We'll need to work out the details—hours, compensation, etc. But on the substance, I'd like you to start working on a concept paper—a piece laying out the issues we want to address about underserved youth and public systems, why these issues are important, and how we plan to address them. Then I'd like your help developing the application we'll use to attract Stoneleigh Fellows. Is that okay with you?"

As Julia began to push her chair away from the small round table where we'd been sitting, I spoke up hurriedly. I needed to say what was on my mind before I lost my nerve.

"Julia, since we're going to work together, I want to tell you that I have kidney disease and am on dialysis." In one sentence, I'd laid my cards on the proverbial table. Didn't all the communications experts say get right to the point?

Julia looked at me for a few seconds as if she hadn't understood what I said. Slowly, she sat back down in her chair across from me.

"Excuse me," she said, her British accent sounding very pronounced. "Oh, Dine. What? When? Tell me."

That afternoon, Julia Dutton became one of a small group of people that I willingly told about my kidney disease and dialysis treatments. I told her the complicated name of my disease, and about the loss of my first kidney, my dialysis schedule, and my current search for a second donor. Julia listened without interrupting and without a hint of pity in her face or body language. She sighed when I finished talking.

"Wow, Dine," she said. "You've been through it."

As I nodded my head in agreement, she continued, "You handle all of this so well. I never would have guessed. You look so beautiful."

I felt a slight jolt of annoyance at Julia's comment about my "beauty." As far as I could see, my appearance had taken quite a hit in the past few years. But I could tell she was sincere.

"Thanks, Julia," I said with a shrug. "I work hard to keep it together."

"Well, I'm sure we can arrange the scheduling," she said getting back to business. "Just let me know if there's ever an issue or if you need anything. And keep me posted about the surgery. I'll be bringing on staff shortly, but I have plenty of work for you. We'll have to do some planning."

We hugged briefly when I stood up to leave. What a relief,

I thought, as I walked out of the Stoneleigh office that day onto 15th and Walnut Streets to hail a cab. Julia Dutton seemed sympathetic and supportive without the drama—just the kind of colleague I needed.

The Amtrak Station at 30th Street was about a mile away from Stoneleigh's office and on another day, I would have walked the distance for the exercise and to prove to myself that I still could. But I was exhausted and instead, stuck out my thumb, hailed a taxi, and jumped in. Despite the February temperatures, sweat trickled down my back— some from the release of anxiety after my meeting and some because I was always sweating. Dialysis seemed to make my menopause symptoms worse. The beautiful clothes I put on that morning were rumpled and limp. I settled into the back seat of the taxi and closed my eyes.

After my meeting at Stoneleigh, I felt strangely hopeful, even when I was back at dialysis sitting in my chair. In a matter of a few weeks, I'd acquired an important, challenging piece of work, and would be bringing home a paycheck that was substantially more than my disability benefits. I would even be taking periodic train trips to Philadelphia for meetings at the Foundation's office. I felt lighter. I wasn't particularly an Emily Dickinson fan, but I thought about her poem that begins *'Hope' is that thing with feathers*. I knew vaguely that the poem is supposed to honor human's capacity for hope in good times and bad. But for me the line also implied that "hope" could fly toward you in one minute then fly wildly away, leaving you in despair, the next. I also thought about civil rights leader Jesse Jackson's famous edict to "keep hope alive."

Was hope my answer? If I could just hold on to this hopeful feeling, would all my dreams come true?

Chapter Thirteen:
HOPE?

Weeks went by and there was still no response from family members to my letter. I thought I'd at least hear from my siblings. But they didn't contact me, and I didn't contact them. I tried not to actively "wait" to hear from someone, filling the time with my foundation work, dialysis, recovering from dialysis, and of course Joe, who was always by my side. Nevertheless, as days passed, my emotions ran the gamut, from anger to hurt, to relief that no one had turned me down yet. I told myself that the silence between me and my siblings wasn't so unusual. Ever since I'd left home way back in 1970, my siblings and I went long periods without talking with each other. I kept trying not to wait.

My sister Linda was the first sibling to respond to my request. She wrote me a letter and turned me down. Linda had been tested back in 2000 during my first search for donors. She was a good match for me. However, she cited her current responsibilities caring for my mother, as the reason she couldn't donate now.

"What if something happens to me," she wrote. "Who will take care of Mommy?" I understood her reasoning. However, Joe was terribly upset and responded with a letter to Linda asking her to reconsider.

"Your sister could die on dialysis," he wrote. "We can figure out the logistics regarding your mom."

But who could disagree with Linda? I certainly couldn't and didn't feel comfortable pushing her anymore.

After Linda's response, the no's seemed to pour in—all, it seemed, with good reasons.

My sister Judy called crying one afternoon to say that her doctor had recommended that she not be a donor. She'd had back surgery as a teenager which had resulted in lifelong back problems.

"I'm sorry, B. The doctor doesn't think it's a good idea," she said through tears.

All I could say was, "I understand, Ju." And I did understand. Why should my sister suffer to give me relief?

My brother Jerry had hernia surgery a few years earlier and needed an additional operation at the site of the original incision. He called one Sunday night to tell me that he'd gotten tested and that we were a match, "but because of this situation with my stomach, B, I can't consider a kidney donation at this time."

Joe and I had talked frequently about respecting my family member's decisions. Both of us, especially me, knew that surgery was a huge step and that there could be any number of good reasons why someone would want to avoid donating one of their kidneys. However, respecting my siblings' decisions, even though they all had good reasons to say no, was easier in theory than in practice. I fantasized about what would have happened had Daddy, the ultimate family man, been around. Could he have pressured one of my siblings to be my donor? Joe kept saying that my sibling's responses felt like "a kick in the gut." I tried to be pragmatic, telling Joe and myself, "No one owes me a kidney, especially if donating is a risk to their own health."

TRANSPLANT: A MEMOIR

~

IN EARLY SPRING 2007, a close relative called to say that they'd been tested. They were a match with me, and willing to be my donor if all the other testing went well. My first emotion, which surprised me, was a bolt of fear from my head to my toes. Was this serious? Was I truly ready to face another transplant? I was also afraid for my potential donor. What if they were injured during the surgery or didn't recover well? Everything had gone okay with Baby Alice, but you never know. However, after I allowed myself to calm down and think about a life without dialysis, my doubts receded to the back of my mind. Joe, my usually sedate husband, shouted out loud when I told him the good news. My mother cried into the telephone. I could almost hear my siblings—Linda, Judy, and Jerry, all breathe a sigh of relief when I told them. While none of them was able to be my donor, they all wanted to see me free of dialysis. As if to seal the deal, my potential donor came to DC and sat through an entire dialysis shift with me. I considered those three hours a "bonding" session.

Julie Trollinger, the transplant coordinator, worked with my donor and me to select a tentative surgery date in June and begin the daunting process of completing all the paperwork and necessary testing. I started a list of things I wanted to take care of around the house and the work I needed to finish for my client before I went into the hospital.

My work at Stoneleigh Foundation was going well. I'd completed the concept paper Julia requested, as well as a draft of the application for attracting Stoneleigh Fellows. I was now helping to assess responses from applicants. Julia completely understood my health issues, but I wanted to stick to our timeline. I wanted to complete every task on my list at least a week before the surgery. I would need time to get my head together before transplant number two. I wanted to spend that last week before the transplant, listening to music and relaxing.

A few weeks before the transplant surgery I had my final exam with Dr. Light, the transplant surgeon. I felt jittery and in need of assurance.

"Dr. Light, you know I lost my first transplant. What happens if this kidney goes bad, too?"

I didn't get assurance from Dr. Light. I got honesty. Since I'd lost my first transplant in 2004, little progress had been made in restoring function to failed kidney transplants.

"We're going to do our best, Ms. Watson," is all that he could say.

In the next day or so, Trollinger called to say that my surgery date and time had been confirmed; that she had spoken with my donor, and everything was in order. We were all set. Until the unthinkable happened. Just a few days later, my donor called to cancel the surgery. They didn't use the term, "cancel," but the word "postpone."

"I need to postpone the surgery due to a scheduling conflict."

I knew they were canceling. The surgery was only two weeks away and they'd known the tentative date for a few months.

As my "donor" stumbled over words trying to explain themselves, a scorching rage bubbled in my throat. I wanted to scream. Why are you laying this shit on me now—a few weeks before the surgery? This is my life we're talking about. But I didn't scream. I gathered my emotions as best I could and whispered into the phone, "I can't talk to you about this now." Then I hung up and called Joe.

"Hi, baby," he answered. "I was just getting ready to call you." This is how Joe answered whenever I called him at work, whether he was getting ready to call me or not. This was a game we played. But I was in no mood for games.

"Joe, I just talked with my donor. They're postponing the surgery."

"What! Are you kidding me?"

"No, I'm not kidding. Please come home."

Later that evening, Joe and I sat curled up together on the living room sofa, as I poured out all my anger, hurt, disappointment, and fear. He was just as angry, disappointed, and scared as I was. We sat in silence for a while letting the new, frustrating reality sink in. Finally, Joe spoke.

"I wish I was compatible with you. I'd give you my kidney tomorrow."

I looked up at my sweet husband. I knew he was telling the truth. I also knew that I'd be back in dialysis the next morning.

~

WHAT NOW?

The question circled in my head for days after my transplant surgery was "postponed." The practical matters were easiest to tackle, and I checked them off as soon as I gathered my energy: call Julie Trollinger so she could alert the hospital, call my family and the few people I'd confided in and give them the news, and let the Stoneleigh Foundation know that I'd be available to work. If anyone at Fresenius knew my surgery had been postponed, they didn't say a word. Of course, my dialysis chair sat waiting for me as usual, arms wide open, as if she knew what had happened.

"Come, sit," she whispered to me. "So what if you'll be here a while longer. It's okay."

Julie Trollinger, the transplant coordinator, was sympathetic on the telephone. "I'm so sorry," she said. "But I have to tell you, Ms. Watson, transplant surgeries fall apart all the time. I spend a lot of time helping patients and families deal with exactly what you're going through."

Trollinger's response seemed wrong to me. "It happens all the time?" I'd read about transplant surgeries falling apart because a donor got cold feet, but that wasn't supposed to happen in my family. "That Hayes family sticks together," is what people always said about us. Even though I knew from experience that the Hayeses didn't come through for each other in every case, I'd been counting on family loyalty in my time of crisis.

Then Julie caught me off guard again. "I spoke to your donor," she said. "They called me a few days ago to let me know what was going on. For confidentiality reasons, I can't tell you the details of our conversation. All I can say is that she feels as badly as you do...."

I interrupted her.

"That can't possibly be true," I said firmly.

"It's true," Julie said, just as firmly. "And I don't think you should give up on this kidney donation. It could still happen. Your donor wants to postpone the surgery, not cancel it."

I knew better. Julie meant well. Part of her job was to keep my spirits up. I appreciated that, but I didn't have her optimism. My options were limited. I had no control over my "donor" and didn't believe the postponement story for a minute. Some days I wanted to scream "liar, liar pants on fire" at the top of my lungs. On other days I tried to put the entire business out of my mind. Joe, on the other hand, called the relative and tried to "talk some sense into them." I asked him not to call them again. Despite my disappointment, I didn't think his pressure was appropriate.

I also had no control over the transplant lists. I hadn't spent a lot of time waiting for a call from one of the transplant centers, but after the experience with my siblings and "donor," I was losing faith that I'd ever get the kidney I needed—from a cadaver or a live human. Is this what I get for daring to be hopeful?

As I think back on those months in 2007, right after plans for my second transplant fell apart, I remember feeling angry, fragile, and insecure. The hope I'd tried hard to cultivate had evaded me. Wherever I went, besides the dialysis center, everyone seemed healthy and whole. Was Fresenius Dupont Circle Dialysis Center the only place I truly belonged? Would I ever have a normal life again, or would I always be a freak with a hole in my arm, who couldn't pee and who needed to have her blood cleansed three times a week? Sometimes, I felt in danger of regressing to my early days at Fresenius when I was so rageful I could barely talk. Of course, Joe, my north star, did what he could to comfort me. Robert loved and cared for me deeply, but I worked hard to hide my pain from him, my mom, and my siblings. They all had their own lives, and I did not want to be a perpetual worry to any of them.

During this time, my work with the Stoneleigh Foundation was one of the things that helped save my sanity. I'd earned that contract with my brain and reputation, regardless of my physical state. The assignments were challenging and relevant, and the fact that Julia and the foundation staff were pleased with my performance did wonders for my frame of mind. Bringing in a regular, substantial paycheck was also gratifying. My heart leaped when every two weeks an envelope from Stoneleigh came through my mail slot. Joe would never let me go wanting, but as the old saying goes, *money is power*. I wanted to contribute more to our household expenses and have my own money to spend as I pleased. A disability check didn't cut it anymore.

But as much as meaningful assignments and generous pay, the sense of independence that came with the work steadied me. The periodic travel back and forth to my beloved hometown, Philly, to meet with Julia and her staff, was a favorite perk. How sweet it was to dress up, carry a handsome tote full of work papers, and take the train up the northeast corridor to an important meeting. I was part of the professional world again, leaving behind, for at least a while, the sights, sounds, and smells of the dialysis world. No one on Amtrak #194 knew that I was a dialysis patient; or that my left arm was wrapped in white gauze to keep blood from seeping out of my fistula and onto my beautiful clothing.

Some of the trips to Philly were just for a day. Others required me to stay over a night or two. Often, I'd stay downtown at the Warwick Hotel on Locust, walking distance to Stoneleigh's office. Even better, sometimes I'd stay with my longtime friend, Alvia, who lived downtown in tony Society Hill. We'd sit laughing and talking into the night. I usually drank more wine than I should, but during those sessions, I felt like a free woman who could do as she pleased. Now and then, because of business travel, I'd miss my regular Monday, Wednesday, and Friday 7:30 a.m. dialysis treatment and need to come in during another shift. The Center staff didn't appreciate my pushing the boundaries of their rigid shift structure but had learned long ago that I was one to challenge the rules if I needed to. While I tried not to be too much of a pain in the ass, I considered the staff's annoyance with me a small price to pay for my improved quality of life.

Also, to help me manage all the ups and downs in my life during this time, I returned to two tools that had served me well in the past: therapy and yoga. I was fortunate to find a woman therapist whose office was within walking distance from my house. She was White, and initially I was reluctant to work with her because of my experience with White therapists when I was in Minnesota. But she had an opening on Thursdays, a non-dialysis day, and took my insurance. Further, during an "informational" appointment, we had a frank discussion about race. I told her that I didn't have a good experience in a women's therapy group led by two White women therapists, and where I was the only Black person in the group.

"Neither therapist saw me clearly nor seemed to know enough about my issues," I said. "My last therapist was Black and frankly, I intended to find another Black provider." The woman didn't blink.

"It's your choice, Dine, but I think I have a broad enough circle of people in my world to be able to understand and work with you on any issue you want to bring to therapy. However, if we work together and you think there's something I'm not understanding, you're going to have to tell me."

Her response was enough for me. I saw this therapist for an hour every Thursday afternoon at 4:00 for about a year. She had a lovely backyard garden where I often sat waiting for my appointment. Those few moments of tranquility among the flowers were a therapy session all by themselves. During my time with her, the therapist encouraged me to value myself and my skills and talents despite my health challenges. She encouraged me to keep a regular yoga and meditation practice as a way of maintaining calm; to pursue my writing goals no matter what was happening with my health; and to be as kind to myself as I could be. My work with her had a lasting effect on me.

In keeping with me being kind to myself, the therapist told me about a small eco-friendly spa, The Stillpoint, that had opened in the neighborhood. I loved the place right away and resumed my yoga practice there on Tuesdays and Fridays at 6:00 p.m. It felt good to stretch my body again, although I had to be careful not to bump the fistula in my left arm. Sometimes my leg muscles cramped when I tried getting into certain poses, I suspected because I needed more water in my system than I was allowed to drink. At The Stillpoint, I also reprised my old habit of regular facials, massages, and mani-pedis—all in the name of taking care of myself.

All these things—therapy, work, yoga, self-care—helped me feel a bit steadier. But on some days the uncertainty about my future and the monotony of dialysis still ate at my nerves. Sometimes I wished I could be more patient or "Zen" about waiting for a cadaver kidney or living donor. Sometimes, I wished I could disappear from dialysis for a few days at a time, like my friend T who sat across the aisle from me when he showed up. I remember the first time I noticed that he'd been absent for a few days.

"Clint," I called across the room after I got settled in my chair, "where's T?" I asked. I could hear the urgency in my voice, but Clint started laughing.

"I don't know where T is, D. You know T be disappearing. He need to get up out of here sometimes."

I was worried about T and decided to press Clint.

"Do you know where he is, Clint? Is T okay?"

Clint shot me a look that seemed part amusement and part exasperation. "D, I told you I don't know where T is. I think he over there at Washington Hospital Center."

Now I was alarmed. T and I had become buddies.

"T's in the hospital? What's the matter with him?"

"I don't know, Miss D," Clint said, shaking his head and still grinning. "Don't get me to lyin'."

That evening, I collected a few sports magazines lying

around my house and headed over to the hospital. Joe offered to go with me, but I turned him down. I wanted T to know that this was a personal visit from a friend, not an errand where I needed my husband to go with me. T looked flabbergasted when I walked into his room.

"Hey, D," T said slowly. "What you doin' here?" T seemed to be slurring his words more than usual, but looked about the same as he did when he came to dialysis.

"I came to see you, T. Clint told me you might be here. What's going on?"

T stared at me and looked confused— shaking his head as if he couldn't believe I was real. "D, I think you the first person to ever visit me in the hospital. I ain't lyin'. But I'm okay," he stuttered. "I just wasn't feeling too good, so I came on in here. That's all."

The whole visit was awkward. I put the sports magazines on a table full of straws and plastic cups and drew the only chair in the room closer to T's bed. For a few minutes we tried to make small talk, but T seemed uncomfortable with my presence as if he couldn't relate to me outside of dialysis. Or maybe he wasn't used to people being kind to him. I couldn't tell, but my visit began to feel like a mistake.

"Well, T," when it seemed that we'd exhausted any possibility of further conversation, "I'm going now. I just wanted to check on you," I said patting his bony hand.

"Okay, now, D," he said, still staring at me as if I were an apparition. "You get home safe now. I'll see you back in dialysis."

On my next dialysis day, I stopped by Clint's chair before getting to my own. "Hey, Clint, I stopped by the hospital to see T the other day. He's doing okay and says he'll be back here in a few days."

This time Clint didn't grin, or just look amused, he burst out laughing, raising his hand to cover his mouth.

"D, D," he said trying to talk between laughs. "You went to the hospital to see T? Ain't nothing more than usual wrong with that man. I coulda' told you that. Ain't nothing wrong with T. He just sick of comin' in here, and he know over at Hospital Center he can get three hots and a cot. They'll keep him over there a few days. Don't waste your time on that fool."

Looking back on that conversation with Clint, I see now that the joke was on me. I wasn't clued into the game T was playing whenever he checked himself into the hospital. But I didn't agree with Clint at all that T was a fool. T had figured out how to make the best out of his difficult circumstances. I admired him. I was struggling to do the same.

~

"Good morning, Ms. Watson."

I looked up from my newspaper to see Dr. Moore standing in front of my chair. I'd almost forgotten that it was Friday and he'd be making rounds.

I was usually glad to see Dr. Moore. We often talked about subjects other than dialysis—like politics and our families. But I recall that on this Friday morning in the fall of 2007, I didn't feel like talking. For some reason, on that day, the weight of another year coming to an end felt particularly heavy. I was still on dialysis and there seemed to be no end in sight.

"Good morning, Dr. Moore," I managed.

"It's time for you to get transplanted, Ms. Watson," he said, unexpectedly. "You're ready. I can tell."

I looked up at Moore wondering if he could see something in my face that I didn't realize was showing. Yes, I was sick and tired of dialysis and still in mourning about the kidney transplant gone awry. Could he read all that in my face or body language? Did he have some "magic" that could get me a kidney simply because I was ready? What about the waiting list and the fact that I had no living donors?

Moore started talking again. You don't interrupt Jack Moore when he's talking.

"The folks from Hopkins have been down to see us about the advances they're making in their Incompatible Kidney Transplant Program (IKTP). The program is led by a surgeon, Bob Montgomery, who's making quite a name for himself. They're doing some pioneering work up there with people who need transplants and have willing donors who are incompatible with them. We aren't offering these programs at Hospital Center yet. We will be, but not yet. I think you and your husband should go up and talk to the folks at Hopkins soon, especially since your other transplant didn't happen. It could make a big difference in how soon you could be off of dialysis."

Dr. Moore had my attention. I had no prospects. I hadn't heard anything from my relative who'd postponed our surgery, which only strengthened my belief that the transplant was canceled and not just postponed. I had almost three years down and possibly seven to go on the transplant list for a cadaver kidney. I wanted to hear about anything that could improve my chances.

Moore took more time than usual with me that morning. Generally, he spent about 10 minutes with each of his patients, quickly reviewing lab results, taking blood pressure readings, answering questions, and doing brief exams. But when his patients needed him, he took the time needed to take care of them.

"Is your husband still willing to give you his kidney?" Moore asked.

"Yes, he is," I answered without hesitation. I lived with a lot of uncertainty, but to paraphrase Oprah, Joe's willingness to be my donor "was one thing I knew for sure."

"Good, good," he responded. Then he went on to tell me that Hopkins could offer two options. First, they used a method called plasmapheresis, where a patient like me could receive a kidney from an incompatible living donor, like Joe. I tried to absorb the complicated information he was giving me, but I must have looked confused.

"Plasmapheresis is similar to dialysis," Moore explained.

Before he could go any further, I rolled my eyes and thought, *Oh, no, not more dialysis. Why does the cure always have to be as bad or worse than the disease?*

Dr. Moore must have seen the look on my face because he held up his hand as if to say, "Just wait a minute and let me finish."

I steeled myself against the back of my chair to hear him out.

Moore explained that plasmapheresis was a process used to remove antibodies from plasma in the blood, just as dialysis was used to remove waste products from the blood. Antibodies, help protect the body from foreign invaders, but could also try to defend the body against a new incompatible kidney and cause the rejection of the new kidney. Plasmapheresis could help to stop the rejection.

"You might need multiple plasmapheresis sessions before and after a transplant to make sure adequate antibodies are removed and your body accepts your husband's kidney. But studies show that patients who receive incompatible kidneys and undergo plasmapheresis keep their organs just as long as those who receive compatible kidneys. If you take this route, you'll likely have to be on higher doses of anti-rejection medication and your

TRANSPLANT: A MEMOIR

spleen might need to be removed since the spleen is the organ that produces antibodies. But this might be an answer for you."

Dr. Moore paused as if to see if I was following him. "Are you okay, Ms. Watson?"

I must have looked a little wan. He reached over and put his hand on my right arm. Moore knew not to jostle my left arm and risk disturbing the dialysis needles.

The doctor was right to ask how I was feeling. I could feel the perspiration making my shirt stick to the back of my chair. At first, I thought my blood pressure was dropping, but none of the nausea or immobilizing leg cramps that usually accompanied such an event was there.

"I'm okay," I said. "I think I got overwhelmed with all the information."

"Are you sure, Ms. Watson? We can continue this another time. I've got plenty of other patients to visit this morning."

I took a quick look around the room. I could see some of Dr. Moore's patients staring in my direction, probably wondering why the doctor was taking so much time at my chair. Further, I was sure Cassandra in the chair next to me could hear every word of my discussion with him. But this morning everyone else could wait. I wanted to hear whatever else Moore had to say.

"I'm feeling okay," I repeated. Could you please tell me what else is available at Hopkins?" I had a ton of questions about plasmapheresis, but I wanted to know the basics about both options so I could talk things over with Joe that evening.

Dr. Moore looked at me with a little impatience but continued. "Well, there's the paired kidney exchange or kidney swap which could also work well for you and your husband."

I already knew that Johns Hopkins was one of the best hospitals in the country. But listening to Dr. Moore, it seemed that they were way out ahead when it came to kidney transplant innovation. Why hadn't I heard about any of these programs? Wasn't it only a few years ago, that Joe and I were racing up I-95 to Hopkins, looking for a miracle that would save my first transplanted kidney?

I forced myself to focus on the information Dr. Moore was providing. The kidney swap or exchange was also difficult to take in. In the swap, Joe and I would be paired with another incompatible pair. I would receive a kidney from the donor in that pair who was compatible with me, and Joe would donate his kidney to the person in the pair he was compatible with. I rolled the doctor's words around in my head to make sure I understood them. His description of the exchange process sounded like one of those probability problems that I was never any good at in high school algebra. Dr. Moore could see the uncertainty on my face.

"Listen, Ms. Watson," he said patting me on my right arm again. "Just think about what I said. Talk it over with your husband later. I'll be back around to take your blood pressure and examine you after you've settled down a bit."

Settle down? Easy for him to say, I thought to myself. I had too much to think about. I pulled my blanket up around my shoulders and slunk down into the chair. Plasmapheresis. Kidney Swaps. The kidney swap option depended on my incompatible husband giving up a kidney. Joe was more than willing to give me a kidney, but I didn't know how he'd feel about giving a kidney to a stranger. I glanced at the clock. It was 10:05. I had twenty-five minutes to go before the tech would be around to unhook me from the machine. I would usually call my mother and talk with her for the rest of the session. But that day I couldn't talk with anyone until I talked with Joe.

Later that evening as we lay in bed, our place of choice for serious discussion, I recounted to Joe my conversation with Dr. Moore, trying my best to keep the details of the medical procedures straight.

"Well, baby," Joe said hoisting himself up on the pillow and looking over at me, "at least we've got options."

I looked back at him and burst out laughing. Suddenly he was cracking up too. As usual, Friday night was our special night, and we had cocooned ourselves in the bedroom to partake. Everything was funnier when we were high. That was one reason we smoked. Sometimes we both needed things to be really funny—hilarious even. Sometimes we needed to be able to laugh really hard.

"Some options, right?" I said to him as I tried to compose myself so I could get the words out.

"Yep," Joe responded, wiping his eyes, and laying back on his pillow. Once Joe started laughing, it wasn't long before tears rolled down his cheeks. Those tears always made me want to laugh even harder.

"So let me get this straight," said Joe, attempting seriousness. "Our options are that I can give you my incompatible kidney, but you would have to have this plasmapheresis treatment and your spleen removed, or I give my kidney to a stranger so you can get a kidney from a stranger."

I didn't answer. Neither of us was laughing at this point. The high seemed to be wearing off for both of us. This was going to be a two-joint night.

"Hm hm hm," Joe grunted. "I guess we have to decide. Let's talk to the Hopkins people, but I think we should look into both things carefully, especially this plasma…however you pronounce it."

Now I was laughing again. For all Joe's smarts and writing

skill, he had trouble pronouncing complicated words. He started laughing again too.

"Seriously though," he continued. "I don't like the idea of you having your spleen removed. I can't believe that."

I believed it. I had three kidneys inside me, all shriveled and useless—the original two in my back and the one my sister gave me which had been tucked into the right side of my stomach. Now I needed a fourth. With all I had been through, I believed anything could happen.

Joe stopped talking. We both lay there in pitch darkness. I knew him well enough to know that he was processing all the information I had given him and would soon have something else to say. I waited.

"One thing's for sure," he said finally, "I'd certainly rather give my kidney directly to you, but if giving it to someone else means you can get a kidney and off dialysis sooner, I'm all for it."

I had known deep down that Joe would respond that way. Still, hearing him say it was such a relief. I closed my eyes. How do I respond to such goodness? Joe always came through for me. As someone who had taken care of herself for as long as I had, I sometimes struggled to accept Joe's goodness. But it just kept coming. I had no words, so I slid my foot over to Joe's side of the bed and rubbed it against his leg. He turned and looked at me. It was one of those moments so tender that it couldn't be sustained. Joe flicked on the light on his night table and got out of bed.

"Let's stop all this talking," he said. "I'm going to roll another joint."

EARLY IN THE FOLLOWING WEEK, while I was sitting in my dialysis chair, I called Hopkins to speak with someone in their IKTP. A nice young lady took my name and number and assured me that someone would get back to me soon. "Soon," I scoffed. I didn't believe her.

A few days later I was walking down Walnut Street in Philadelphia, feeling pretty good. My meeting at the Stoneleigh Foundation had gone well and ended earlier than I'd anticipated. I'd spent the extra time walking west on Walnut Street and poking around in a few of my favorite Philly shops. I planned to reach Rittenhouse Square at 18th and Walnut and rest on a bench for a while before heading to the train back to DC and an evening dialysis session.

As I stood on the corner just across the street from the Square, my cell phone began to ring. I could hear the ringtone—a sweet doorbell chime—but I couldn't put my hand on the phone itself. I was sure it had fallen to the bottom of my tote under the legal pads, wallet, make-up case, reading material, and other stuff that I carried around, especially when I was traveling on business. As usual, I had forgotten to put the damn thing in the side pocket of my bag so I could easily get to it. I fumed to myself, *in my next life, I want to be more organized, and, oh yeah, not have kidney disease.*

Wow. How many rings did I set for this phone? After what seemed like an entire minute, the phone was still ringing, and I couldn't put my hands on it. I was starting to feel a little self-conscious, since, in my opinion, nothing looks tackier than a woman rummaging around in her pocketbook as she walks down the street. Who could be calling me so insistently—Stoneleigh? Joe? Robert? Only a few people had my cell phone number. Finally, I felt the leather case that held my little black flip phone.

"Hello, Dine Watson," I said in my best professional voice, masking all the frustration of digging for my phone.

"Hello, Ms. Watson?"

"Yes," I responded, tentatively. I didn't recognize the person on the other end of the line. Besides, I could barely hear them over the clamor of Walnut Street's midday traffic.

"Ms. Watson, this is Dr. Montgomery from Johns Hopkins. How are you doing?"

I stopped so suddenly in the middle of 18th street that I caused the woman walking behind me stumbled into me. She gave me an annoyed, side-eyed glance as she moved to my left. Ordinarily, I would have apologized to her, but I was stunned. Dr. Robert Montgomery, genius transplant surgeon, was on my cell phone, sounding very casual and friendly.

"I'm doing well today, Dr. Montgomery," I managed to say. It was true. I was doing well. I was in my beloved Philly and not yet in DC hooked up to a dialysis machine. Yes, I was well.

"How are you?" I asked him in return, as I hurried out of the middle of the street and plopped down on a bench near the edge of Rittenhouse Square.

What could Dr. Montgomery want? He was head of the Incompatible Kidney Transplant Program at Hopkins. Why would he be calling me himself? I was about to find out.

"I understand that you might be interested in our transplant program. I've seen your file and I think you and your husband should come in and talk with us," he said as calmly as if he was giving me a recommendation on where to have lunch. But Montgomery wasn't recommending lunch. He had taken the time to call me himself to talk about my kidneys. I was impressed.

The good doctor went on to explain that according to my labs, I was in great health for someone who had been on dialysis for almost four years, and just as important, I had a healthy, willing donor, my husband, who wasn't my blood type. He encouraged me to think about starting the evaluation process for Hopkins' kidney transplant programs designed specifically for incompatible pairs.

I was tired that evening after I got home from my late dialysis treatment. However, I was anxious to talk with Joe about my conversation with Montgomery. Based on what we'd learned from Drs. Montgomery and Moore, both of Hopkins' transplant approaches had pros and cons. Getting me transplanted and off dialysis as soon as possible was a priority, but neither Joe nor I wanted to take unnecessary chances. With the plasmapheresis process, it seemed we could move ahead more quickly since the only people required would be me and Joe. However, going through a dialysis-like process while still receiving my regular dialysis treatments was unappealing. And the possibility of having my spleen removed to encourage my body to accept Joe's incompatible kidney sounded risky. On the other hand, who knew how long it would take to find a compatible "pair" so that we could participate in the kidney exchange program? I could still be on dialysis for a significant amount of time before a match was found.

In the end, we decided to go up to Hopkins to be evaluated for both approaches.

"We'll take things step by step, making decisions as we go along," Joe said. "That's the only thing that makes sense, especially now that both of us have skin in this game."

"Literally," I replied, laughing at my attempt at a joke.

"Well, I meant my wedding vows, in sickness and in health," Joe said with a serious tone.

"I know you did. I did, too. We promised," I responded.

At that point, Joe started to sing, in his off-key tone, the words to the Temptation's song "Promise."

"Please stop singing, Joe," I begged. "I'll go dig out the CD if you want me to."

At this point were both laughing. But there was nothing laughable about this tune. "Promise" is one of the most earnest and heartfelt songs about romantic commitment ever written. Joe and I had fallen in love with the song after we slow-danced to it at a friend's wedding. Ever since then, "Promise" was the song we called on to remind us of the promises we'd made to each other.

Chapter Fourteen:
HOPING AND WAITING

In March 2008, Joe and I began driving up and down I-95 between DC and Johns Hopkins in Baltimore so both he and I could complete the testing necessary for the transplant program. When we could, we arranged our appointments on the same day. When same-day appointments weren't possible, we drove up to Baltimore together anyway, rearranging dialysis and work schedules as necessary.

It wasn't lost on us that in 2004, the year we married, we were making the same trek from DC to Hopkins trying to save my first transplanted kidney. Now four years later we were gambling on Hopkins again, hoping this time for a better outcome. Sometimes the testing was tedious and took all day. But Joe and I found ways to make the days bearable, sometimes even fun. On breaks between appointments, we'd walk or drive around Baltimore looking at neighborhoods, architecture, and places we wanted to revisit under other circumstances. We also discovered Sabatino's, an old-school restaurant in Little Italy that we loved so much, we made it our official lunch stop.

During a day of appointments at Hopkins, Joe and I met Dr. Montgomery, the doctor who had called me in Philadelphia. Montgomery, who would be our surgeon if we had the transplant surgery at Hopkins, looked nothing like I'd imagined. In all my years of dealing with nephrologists, they had all looked the part—buttoned-up, clean-shaven, and conservative. Not this doctor. Robert Montgomery had long, slicked-back hair, a handlebar mustache, and wore cowboy boots. He had a quick smile, a hearty laugh, and seemed to have absolutely no pretense. We met with Montgomery in a small examination room in the middle of a busy clinic. He pulled two stools into the room and drew the white curtain around us for privacy. The doctor then folded his tall frame onto another stool and sat with his hands folded in his lap, as if he had nothing to do all day but talk with us and answer our questions.

By the time we saw Montgomery, he had reviewed both Joe's and my test results. I was impressed with how clearly and honestly he spoke about our situation even if I was disappointed with the bottom line of his remarks. Not only was Joe not my blood type, but our tests showed that my body produced significant antibodies against his tissue. In other words, both our blood and tissue types were incompatible. Therefore, he explained that Joe would not be a good donor for me using the plasmapheresis option. Because of our two areas of incompatibility, I would probably need more anti-rejection medication after the transplant than he thought prudent. Montgomery must have seen in my records that while I was on immunosuppressants with my first transplant, I developed pre-cancerous growths.

"It's important that you're not overly immunosuppressed," Montgomery said.

Joe and I looked at each other and frowned. By this time in our marriage, I could read Joe's mind and knew exactly what he was thinking, *I know we didn't drive up here for this doctor to tell us there's nothing you can do!* But that wasn't the case at all.

TRANSPLANT: A MEMOIR

"We should talk about the other option, our paired donation approach," added Montgomery, breaking through the obvious tension in the little room.

Based on my earlier conversation with Dr. Moore, I already knew the basics of the paired donation. However, Montgomery had more information about how the approach worked. He explained that the names of donors and recipients, along with their blood and tissue types, were fed into a computer database to find appropriate matches.

"The more pairs in the database, the more potential matches." Montgomery clasped his hands together in what seemed like delight. He also explained that Hopkins was now receiving and including in their database, recipient/donor pairs from other transplant centers, which provided a larger pool and therefore greater opportunity for matching and transplanting.

"In fact," he said, "I'm advocating for a national program to facilitate this pairing process since this could increase the number of kidneys available for donation."

The more Montgomery talked, the more my breath quickened. Maybe this paired exchange was the way to go. Joe had already said he was willing to give his kidney to a stranger if it meant I could get a transplant. So why couldn't this work for us? I grabbed Joe's hand in excitement.

"So, are you recommending we go with the paired exchange, doctor?" As usual, my journalist husband wanted to get down to specifics.

"We're certainly going to add you to the database immediately, but I must tell you that you shouldn't expect to get to the front of the exchange line right away. You, Ms. Watson, are 'O Positive' and require an 'O' donor. Since 'O' donors are universal donors and can give to anyone, those kidneys are in high demand. Also, since you've already had a transplant, your body has built up antibodies against any new kidney. We'll have to find a donor for you where the sensitivity is less of a problem. We'll do our best, but it could be a while."

As Montgomery began to exit the exam room, I blurted out the question that I'd been too scared to ask.

"Doctor, how long does it usually take to match an exchange pair?"

"Well, it can take anywhere from one month to two years," Montgomery said, "probably closer to the two-year mark for you because of your blood type." He then waved goodbye and exited the room, his cowboy boots clicking against the tile floor.

Joe and I stayed behind in the examining room for a few minutes to assess our situation. Neither of us was ecstatic. One of the transplant options we'd been considering was now off the table. The other option could still require a considerable waiting period. However, I could tell that Joe was coming to the same conclusion as I was. I'd already been on dialysis for three and one-half years. Even if it took two years, the maximum time Montgomery cited, for Hopkins to find an exchange pair for us, I would still have been on dialysis for a shorter period than the average time I could wait for a cadaver kidney. And I would still be accumulating time on the waiting list for a cadaver kidney at three hospitals.

"I think this kidney exchange option is the best we can do right now," Joe said.

"I'll take it," I responded.

Although nothing much was going to change immediately, signing on to Hopkins' paired exchange program renewed my hope. After meeting Montgomery, I read everything I could find out about him on the internet. Not only was the doctor a brilliant, pioneering kidney transplant surgeon, but he also seemed to be a fabulous human being. Montgomery's colleagues described him as "someone who thinks outside of the box," and who will "step up and take risks for his patients." He'd also spent time in remote areas of West Africa doing public health medicine.

I don't remember how I first learned that Montgomery was engaged to marry opera singer Denyce Graves, but the news gave me goosebumps. The surgeon who could potentially perform my kidney transplant was engaged to a Black woman. I read in a newspaper article that he described her as the most beautiful woman he'd ever seen. Reading this, I felt excited that Montgomery just might be a doctor who would see me, a Black woman, as a human being and not just a body— someone who deserved to be treated with care. If I was going to have another transplant, I wanted Montgomery to be the surgeon.

While there were still no guarantees, after the meeting with Montgomery, both Joe and I understood that we had some semblance of a plan, and possibly, a more favorable timeframe to hold on to. We decided not to tell our families, not even our children, about the Hopkins' program. The only expectations we'd have to manage would be our own.

The hopefulness I felt from the Hopkins/Montgomery connection also seemed to energize me. I felt stronger. For the first time since I'd started treatment, I dared to think about life after dialysis. This new vitality made me wonder how much my fatigue and weariness over the past three years had been due to the psychological impact of being on dialysis. Thinking about the power of "hope" I read, for the first time, the entire Dickinson poem and not just the title. I was struck by the first stanza:

Hope is the thing with feathers
That perches in the soul,

And sings the tune without the words,
And never stops at all

What would happen if I allowed a bit of hope to perch in my soul? I didn't know what would happen. I had never been a particularly hopeful person. But I wanted to find out.

During the summer of 2008, I decided to put my newfound hopeful energy to the test. I had plenty of inspiration. That summer, the entire country was talking about "hope" either positively or scornfully, depending on whether they supported the presidential candidacy of Senator Barack Obama, who used the word as a theme in his campaign. I was politically savvy enough to know that Obama's theme was mainly rhetoric. However, the fact that a Black man had secured the Democratic nomination and could become president of the United States, lifted my spirits and added to my hopeful energy quotient.

In July, I decided to spend some of my energy "chits" on a trip to Chicago, accompanying Joe to the five-day Unity Journalist Convention, an every four-year gathering that brought together the National Association of Black Journalists, the National Association of Hispanic Journalists, the Asian American Journalists Association, and the Native American Journalists Association. Because 2008 was an election year, Democratic presidential nominee, Barack Obama would address the more than ten thousand journalists of color expected to attend the meeting. How could I miss that? To me, going to the convention felt like a good omen. On Sunday, July 27th, I sat among thousands of journalists of color, and listened to Barack Obama, possibly the next president of the United States, discuss how, if elected, he planned to address issues of concern to US citizens of color. Being at the Unity conference made me feel hopeful about my future and the future of the country.

Of course, to be in Chicago for five days meant I'd had to arrange two dialysis sessions at a Fresenius Center near my hotel. I also had to try and adhere to my other requirements for being out in the world: 1) no matter how tempting the food or drink, stick to the dialysis diet; 2) take an afternoon nap to conserve my precious energy and just as important as the first two requirements; 3) always wear long sleeves to cover the bulging fistula in my left arm.

Fresh off my attendance at the Unity Conference, I accepted another consulting assignment. Bathing in a sea of accomplished journalists, many of whom were African American and my peers in age, had made me feel anxious and doubtful about my place in the professional world. Yes, I'd been an executive at a leading social policy organization, but the operative words were "had been." I told myself that I should be making more of a mark in the world, and the small contract with the Stoneleigh Foundation didn't seem like enough. I knew I needed to take care of myself, but I also felt a growing urgency to be more productive. If indeed I was moving closer to resuming my normal life, I wanted to hit the ground running.

The consulting assignment, with the Foundation for Child Development, was to conduct a year-long study of the Pre-K for All DC Initiative in Washington DC. The study would require me to observe pre-kindergarten programs in DC and interview key people across the political, financial, educational, and community sectors to determine how well the initiative advanced the cause of universal pre-kindergarten in the District. This work seemed exactly what I needed. First, pre-kindergarten education was a major policy issue across the country and DC had one of the most-watched campaigns. My study of the District's efforts could make a major contribution to the discussion. Second, carrying out the study in DC would put me directly in touch with many of DC's movers and shakers. I'd been on dialysis for most of the time I'd been in DC and hadn't made many contacts beyond Joe's friends and colleagues at *The Washington Post*. Frankly, I wanted to establish my *own* reputation in DC—a town where everybody seems to be somebody. I felt certain I could handle this new project in addition to my Stoneleigh work and keep myself relatively well. I'd schedule my interviews on Tuesdays and Thursdays—non-dialysis days—and conduct as many as practical by telephone. Most of the work, writing the report, would be done while sitting at my trusty wooden desk or in my dialysis chair if necessary.

I had no choice but to tell my new client, The Foundation for Child Development, about the possibility of a major surgery that could interrupt my availability. They didn't seem too concerned, so I decided not to let the possibility worry me either. Joe supported my decision to take on the additional work.

"Baby, you know what you can handle," he told me. "I'll back whatever you want to do."

Truth be told, Joe, a diligent worker himself, admires industrious, accomplished people. If I was okay, he was fine with me pushing myself.

And that's exactly what I did, push myself. I took monthly train trips up to Philadelphia for work on my original contract with the Stoneleigh Foundation, interviewed DC Council members and other leaders across the District for the Pre-K initiative evaluation, and wrote furiously at my desk. I was often exhausted, but I was also quite satisfied to be in the world exercising my mind and talent, not just sitting in a dialysis chair trying to hold my ailing body together.

Being busy made me more careful, not less, about taking

care of myself. I worked even harder to adhere to the dialysis diet and counted on my weekly therapy visits, yoga, and meditation practices to help keep my mind and body as fit as possible. I didn't want any weakness, mental or physical, to interfere with my work. I was eager to show myself, as much as others, what I was capable of despite my illness. Sometimes, when I stopped to think, I was amazed by what I accomplished.

Still, no matter how much activity I'd piled onto my plate, or what else was going on in my mind, I was always listening, waiting, and hoping for a call about a compatible donor. I was still on transplant lists at the University of Penn, Johns Hopkins, and Washington Hospital Center for a cadaver kidney. But the call I wanted was from the Hopkins' program. That call would mean three things of utmost importance to me: first, I'd have a live donor, which all the data said was a better option than a cadaver; second, Dr. Montgomery would be my surgeon, something I was convinced would make a positive difference in the outcome of the surgery, and third, my husband and best pal, Joe would be involved in the four-way kidney swap—something that gave me a great deal of confidence and comfort.

∽

BY THE END of the summer of 2008, I had not heard from Hopkins or the other hospitals, but I got an email I wasn't expecting—from a woman named Marty. Marty knew all my trials with FSGS and dialysis because she was the sister of a good friend. Maybe her email should not have been as unexpected as it was. Late in 2007, Marty had mentioned to me that she might be interested in being my kidney donor. At the time, I thanked her kindly but did not give a lot of serious thought to her comments. During my time on dialysis, a few friends had made the same offer, but in the end, never got around to completing even the preliminary testing. Besides, after my experience with the relative who'd said she'd be my donor only to opt out at the last minute, I was from Missouri, the "show me state" when I heard such talk. Marty was a nurse, and I knew her well enough to believe she wouldn't make such an offer without thinking it through first. But the sister of a friend wanting to give me a kidney? How likely was that to happen? However, when I heard from Marty again in 2008, I paid attention.

One evening while I was at my desk working, I noticed an email from Marty. After reading her message I ran into the living room and shouted up the steps to Joe.

"Joe, listen to this. Marty is serious about being my donor." After reminding him of who Marty is, I read him this email from her:

"Just wanted to bring you up to date. We did go to the University of Penn hospital today. So far so good. There's nothing obvious in my medical history that would rule me out. They drew blood and gave me a container for a 24-hour urine, should we be a good match. While we're waiting for those results, I'll go ahead and gather some other medical records. I'm not sure what the next step will be, but I'll be sure to keep you in the loop."

"Can you believe this?" I asked, still shouting.

"Well, I think we have to believe it," Joe said, swinging his chair around from his desk. "Marty seems clear. She's moving forward with this thing."

"Sure, seems so," I said, beginning to use my "inside" voice.

I stared at Joe and he at me without saying a word. I knew we were thinking the same thing. He spoke first. "Look, babe, let's not get too excited about this. We've been disappointed before."

For a moment I didn't say anything. I knew he was right.

"Okay, okay, I know," I said shrugging my shoulders. It's too early anyway. We don't even know if she's a match…, but can't we be a little excited? This woman thinks I'm worthy of her kidney. Isn't that something to be excited about?"

Joe stood up out of his chair and opened his arms wide and I stepped in for a hug.

"Get a little excited if you want to. Honestly, I'm a little excited myself. It's always good to have options. And if things don't work out with Marty, we still have Hopkins, right?"

I sighed and answered, "right."

Joe and I added "Marty" to our list of calls to wait for, while trying to mute our hope and excitement that the sister of my friend could end up being my donor. However, when Joe and I learned from Marty that based on initial testing, she and I had the same O-positive blood type, we allowed ourselves some optimism.

"Oh, what good news, what good news," Joe said hugging me. "Maybe this 'hope' business works."

"Maybe," I said hesitantly. "Remember, there still has to be some tissue typing to make sure my body will accept her kidney. And I know from the time Baby Alice was my donor that Marty still has to undergo lots of other tests to make sure she doesn't have any underlying conditions and is healthy enough to donate."

Joe shook his head. He understood. But try as we might, we couldn't keep ourselves from speculating and getting excited about what this news from my friend's sister could mean.

"Since Marty's in the Philly area, it might make sense to have the surgery at Penn and not at Hopkins or Washington Hospital Center."

"Maybe you could stay with Rob while I'm in the hospital. He lives right across the bridge from Penn."

"If this all works out, we should have a big dinner before the surgery so that our and Marty's family can meet," I said. But I was getting ahead of myself.

We were devastated when Marty called one afternoon to tell us that she would have to withdraw her offer to be my donor.

"I'm so sorry, Dine," she said, sounding devastated herself. "I've been having a lot of back pain over the past several months. I didn't think it was anything that would interfere with my donation, but my GP thinks I will likely have back surgery soon. He recommends that I not undergo kidney surgery at this time. I'm so sorry."

Years later, Marty would tell me tearfully that yes, back in 2008, her doctor had recommended she not go through with the transplant, but that there was more to the story.

"When it was time for me to have further testing to determine whether or not I would be a good candidate for the transplant, my family, in particular my children, got cold feet and didn't want me to go through with the surgery. My back was an issue, but I wish I had pushed harder to find out how much of an issue it would be. It was very hard for me to tell you I couldn't be your donor and I've felt bad about it ever since."

Joe and I were stunned at Marty's disclosure and assured her that in 2008, we'd been grateful for her offer even though she hadn't been able to go through with the donation. I remember at the time saying something to Marty that I thought might make her feel better. I also remember that after her call, Joe and I sat on the sofa and cried. We'd been here before and neither of us could immediately find words to comfort the other.

∼

TRANSPLANT: A MEMOIR

ONE MONDAY IN NOVEMBER, I noticed that T wasn't in his chair. He and I had become good friends ever since I visited him in the hospital. After he got over the shock of my visit, T bragged to anyone at dialysis who would listen.

"Do you know that D came to visit me in the hospital," he'd say grinning as he tried hard to get the words out. "I looked up and there she was."

The staff and patients would look at me and then back at T inquisitively as if they were wondering, what in the world is going on? I'd look back at them, slyly as if something was going on between T and me. And there was—friendship. I'd brought him an Obama baseball cap back from the Chicago Convention which he wore every day he came to dialysis. I have to say, as banged up as T's body was, he sure looked good in that red cap.

When T hadn't shown up by the end of the week, I tried not to worry. Maybe he was taking a few "mental health" days away from dialysis or was back in the hospital. Finally, I decided to inquire about him.

"Hey, Clint," I called across the room like I was calling to a neighbor over the back fence. "Where's T?"

Clint jerked his head up from a nap, looked at me, and shook his head.

"D, do I look like T's keeper? I have no idea where he is. Maybe over there in the hospital again. Why you always worryin' 'bout that man," he said before closing his eyes and turning his head away from me.

That evening, I called Washington Hospital Center to see if T had been admitted, but the operator politely told me "We don't have anyone here by the name of Theodore Wooley."

By the following Friday, T had been missing from dialysis for two weeks. When Dr. Moore arrived for his usual Friday rounds, I was determined to ask him about my friend. When he got to my chair, I waited until he had finished examining me and asked if he knew where T was.

Dr. Moore frowned and shifted his weight from one foot to the other. "I don't know, Ms. Watson," he said shaking his head in what looked like resignation. "I haven't been notified that he's at Hospital Center. Maybe the social worker knows something."

Where could T be? He was homeless, in poor physical health and unless he was getting treatment elsewhere, had missed over two weeks of dialysis. How can anybody on dialysis survive on the street or even in a shelter? Is he getting enough to eat? On some days, I'd been slipping a few dollars into his pocket, but if he didn't come in, I couldn't help him.

When I saw the social worker, I asked if she knew of T's whereabouts. She tossed her hair and looked exasperated. "I don't know where he is, Ms. Watson. We've tried to help Mr. Wooley. His sister is willing to take him in, but he doesn't want to live with her. She hasn't heard from him. He'd rather be on the street. We've done all we can."

Joe also hadn't seen him on his usual bench in Lafayette Square.

Weeks went by with no sight of T at the dialysis center and no mention of him by the staff or even Clint. One morning towards the end of the year, I arrived at the Center to find a strange woman sitting in T's chair. I knew I'd never see him again.

Fresenius Dialysis Center was quieter for me without T. The room was still filled with the noise of patient chatter, cart wheels rolling in the aisles, or someone crying out in pain. Due to his stroke-induced speech impediment, T had rarely added to the noise in the room anyway. It was actually Clint's "noise" that was missing—his boisterous conversations with T, and his silly clowning when I walked by his chair. Clint was also much more subdued without his sidekick, T, there to laugh at his antics. I can't say that I missed Clint's "noise," but I did feel sorry for him. We never talked about it, but I think he missed his friend T. I did too.

Apart from T's absence and Clint's quietness, my dialysis treatments went on as usual. Joe still drove me to the Center in the morning as we listened to NPR. The blood, the needles, and my struggles with the diet remained the same. I still juggled my treatment schedule when I needed to accommodate my work. The Center staff still didn't like the liberties I took but found a way to accommodate me.

However, the more time passed, the more toll the treatments took on my body. I developed an infection in my fistula, the access used for my dialysis treatments. An arteriovenous fistula like the one I had in my arm is considered the "gold standard" of dialysis accesses because they have a lower tendency to clot and get infected. Nevertheless, one morning, I awoke feeling feverish. My left arm and hand were swollen, sore, and warm to the touch, and a nasty-looking substance was oozing from my fistula. I remember a dialysis technician looking at my arm, winching, and calling Nurse Margaret to have a look. The nurse immediately called my doctor to prescribe a course of antibiotics. When I asked Nurse Margaret what caused the infection, she said gravely,

"Well, you have to make sure you're keeping your access clean by washing it with soap every day, and you have to make sure you don't sleep on it. But honestly, Ms. Watson, any opening in the skin, like the repeated needle pokes used in dialysis, can be an entry point for infection." Then Nurse Margaret raised her voice a bit and said, "Ms. Watson, being on dialysis affects your immune system and your ability to fight off infection. This is serious. You could die from an infection like this. Make sure you fill that prescription and start taking the medication right away. We'll keep an eye on it here, but if it doesn't get better within a few days you may have to be hospitalized."

The look on Nurse Margaret's face told me something I had always suspected. Despite her tough exterior, she cared about her patients. But her concern about my arm scared me. The infection began to clear in a few days but left me feeling extremely vulnerable. I realized that no matter how well I followed the rules, or how much "hope" I carried in my heart, the longer I was on dialysis the more chance that some small bacteria would enter my body and if they so pleased, kill me. Looking at my swollen, red arm, I couldn't help but wonder if my luck might be running out.

I began to feel sick to my stomach after every treatment. Not the full-on body cramps and vomiting I experienced with a blood pressure drop (although I still had those episodes from time to time). This was a nauseous feeling that settled into the pit of my stomach after dialysis and stayed for a few hours. My doctor prescribed Nexium, but I preferred an indulgence from my childhood. After dialysis, I'd stop at a tiny, overcrowded, grocery store on the corner of 16th and T to buy a $.50 bag of pretzels. I'd grown up on pretzels, but as an adult had eaten them sparingly because of their high salt and carbohydrate content. Now the salt helped settle my stomach for a while.

In March 2009, Joe received a letter from the transplant coordinator at Hopkins' Department of Surgery advising him that his status in the Kidney Paired Donation database remained "active." The letter also requested his permission to enter our names and tissue typing information into the databases of three new Kidney Paired Donation programs with whom they had recently partnered. The last line of the letter read, "We remain very optimistic that these collaborative efforts will increase your and your recipient's chances for a transplant in the very near future."

Of course, we signed and returned the Medical Release of Information form the same day. Referring to the language in the letter, Joe commented facetiously, "Me and Hopkins probably have different definitions for *the very near future*. For me, the near future is next week. They're probably talking about next year."

Joe and I did our best to keep each other calm. At least once every few days one of us would dredge up that old folk saying that things happen when they are supposed to happen. I'm not sure that I believed the old saying, though. Was I supposed to wait this long for a kidney? Nevertheless, there was nothing to do but wait, hope, and then take what 2009 sent our way.

We waited but jumped every time the telephone rang. Later in March, while we were having dinner in the kitchen, Robert called with surprising personal news.

"Ma, I'm going to be a father," my thirty-eight-old son said softly into the phone.

I'd heard him but shouted back, "What did you say?" If he was going to give me such surprising news, I wanted him to speak up and claim his statement.

"I'm going to be a father, Mom," Rob shouted back at me.

I certainly hadn't been expecting this news. In fact, to my knowledge, Robert hadn't been serious about that many women. I wasn't sure that I would have grandchildren.

"What a shock," I said to Joe after I got off the telephone. "I'm going to be a grandmother."

Joe looked up from the newspaper he was reading at the kitchen counter and asked in a tone of disbelief. "What? That was Robert?" Joe then started in with the questions of his trade, Who, What, When? "I want details."

I laughed and said, "I don't have any details. I didn't even know Rob was dating anyone. All he told me is that I'm going to be a grandma and he's bringing the young lady to meet us in a few weeks. By the way, it's going to be 'Nana Dine' for me."

To which Joe responded, "You know this is going to be my grandbaby too, even if she's not my blood. I'll be Papa Joe."

I wouldn't have expected anything less from Joe, but I loved hearing him say this.

"Aren't you happy?" Joe asked, this time letting go of the newspaper altogether. When my husband put a newspaper down to have a conversation, I knew he was serious.

"Yes, I'm happy. I'd love to have a grandbaby, boy or girl. But this new life gives me something else to worry about. What if I pass my FSGS on to the baby? There's so much unknown about this disease. I'm told that FSGS is not hereditary and so far, so good, with Robert. But it may have a genetic component. FSGS can jump around in families and even skip generations."

Joe reached across the kitchen counter and hugged me. "Come on, Dine. You're borrowing trouble. The baby's not even here yet. Enjoy this news and don't worry so much."

Of course, Joe was right. He often is.

A few months later as I sat at my desk working, I heard the phone ring and saw that the call was from Washington Hospital Center. I was surprised to hear Julie Trollinger, the Hospital Center's transplant coordinator on the other end of the line. I hadn't spoken to Julie in months.

"Hi, Ms. Watson," Julie said quickly. "How are you? A cadaver kidney has just become available that's a match for you. I'm calling to see if you're interested."

What? A potential donor?

"Julie," I said, speaking quickly myself. "I wasn't expecting this. I didn't think I'd accumulated enough time on the transplant list."

"Ms. Watson," she responded, "that's why we give people average wait times. We can't predict when a compatible kidney will become available. If you're interested, you need to let me know right away and get to the hospital quickly."

My head was spinning, Was I interested? With the Hopkins live donor option in the picture, I'd almost forgotten about the transplant lists. I knew a kidney from a live donor was better, but maybe this cadaver kidney would be my only shot.

"Julie, please give me a chance to talk with Joe and get back to you in a few minutes."

"Okay, Ms. Watson, but let me give you some information that might be helpful. The donor is male and in his seventies. That's on the upper end of the kidneys we accept for transplant. You should consider that information, talk with your husband and get back to me as soon as possible."

By the time I contacted Joe at his office, I knew I didn't think a seventy-year-old cadaver kidney was best for me.

"I don't want to seem ungrateful," I told him.

"Don't worry about that, babe. This is your life. I don't blame you for feeling this way. I don't think Julie will either. That kidney will get a good home, just not in your body."

When I called Julie back, I was careful to express my gratitude first and then tell her my decision. She was very understanding.

"Ms. Watson, I get it. If I were you, I'd probably make the

same decision. This kidney is a little old for you and you want to give yourself the best chance possible for a healthy life. I think you and your husband are right to wait on Hopkins."

That's exactly what we did. Wait.

Joe and I went camping in the Shenandoah mountains that summer. We were driving to our campsite on July 3rd when Rob called to say that his partner Kim was in labor, and they were headed to Pennsylvania Hospital. We considered turning around and heading to Philadelphia before reminding ourselves that Rob and Kim were both grown and, with the help of the doctors, could handle the situation.

"Call us if you need to," I told Rob.

On that camping trip, I surprised myself by, in my diminished condition, hiking five miles through the woods. I attributed my strength and endurance to my daily yoga practice. Truth be told however, I was faint with thirst by the time I finished the hike and had to nap and suck on ice cubes for the rest of the afternoon to recover.

I can't remember the day in August when we got a call from the coordinator at Hopkins telling us they'd found a compatible donor for me and a compatible recipient for Joe. I also don't remember any great rejoicing by Joe or me. While we both had a great deal of confidence in Hopkins and our ponytailed surgeon, we'd been disappointed many times and didn't want to get too far ahead of ourselves. I'd be lying if I didn't admit to exhaling a bit at the thought of the transplant surgery, but I tried hard to be practical.

"Let's wait until we get something in writing from Hopkins before we get too excited," I said to Joe.

An email titled "Pre-operative Appointment Letter and other Educational Items" arrived on September 8 giving us the date and time of our surgery—September 22nd, at 5:30 a.m.—and a list of preoperative instructions.

"Can we get excited now?" Joe asked jokingly.

But I was still cautious. I knew that even scheduled surgery could be postponed for any number of reasons. I shivered at the thought of how my first transplant was delayed for three weeks after I got an infection in the hospital.

"Okay, okay, yes, we can get excited," I said, shouting, "finally" at the top of my voice.

∽

WHEN I REALIZED that the time between September 8 to September 22 was exactly two weeks, I would have wet my pants if I could pee. Joe and I had exactly fourteen days to not just take care of all the medical business Hopkins required, but to handle whatever personal business needed taking care of before having major surgery. Both of us had professional work to tie up. I also prepared and froze several chicken and vegetarian dinners that we could pop into the microwave when we returned home from the hospital.

We each called our closest friends and relatives to give them the details. Everyone seemed ecstatic and relieved, although Rob and Kim, while happy for me, were preoccupied with their new baby girl, Naomi Grace.

I, of course, had the task of saying goodbye to my dialysis community forever—that is if the gods of luck favored me, and the transplant was successful. I had not kept anyone at the Center abreast of my transplant activities. Although no one had said anything to me, I was sure at least some of the staff were aware of all my efforts since they were responsible for sending my blood samples off to the various hospitals. But the patients knew nothing about my impending surgery. What was I supposed to say?

I wasn't concerned about the people on my shift that I only knew to speak to casually. I did worry about saying goodbye to my row-mate Cassandra and my "buddy" Clint across the aisle, both of whom I'd talked to about transplants. Would they think I was bragging? Would they be happy for me or think I was making a big mistake? Maybe they wouldn't care at all.

I waited until the day before my surgery to say goodbye. On Monday, September 21st, after my technician unhooked me from the machine, I walked over to Cassandra's chair.

"San," I said, using her nickname, "I'm having transplant surgery tomorrow. So, I want to say goodbye. Fingers crossed for me, okay?"

At first, Cassandra looked confused. I could almost see the wheels rewinding in her head until she remembered our earlier conversation about me "thinking about" having a transplant. Cassandra didn't cross her fingers, but said, "Okay, girl, good luck," in a tone that sounded dispassionate to me.

I might have bent over and hugged her, but I didn't want to disturb the needles in her arm. I also didn't have on a mask and didn't want to get too close to her dialysis access. So, I just waved, gathered my things, and walked toward the nurses' station.

Most of the staff knew about my surgery. Everyone took turns wishing me the best. I even got a warm smile from Nurse Margaret which I returned as warmly. She'd taken good care of me. My favorite technician, David, the handsome Jamaican, came around from behind the desk, hugged me, and slipped his email address into my hand.

I had to pass Clint's chair to get to the Center door. He was sleeping. As I stood wondering if I should wake him, I remembered my early days at Fresenius when, as I walked by his chair, he would call out to me with some ridiculous comment. I'd hated to walk by him and frankly almost hated him back then. Watching him now made me think of my friend T and wonder if he was dead or alive. I touched Clint's free arm lightly.

He stirred, blinked his red eyes open, and stared at me as if he were trying to figure out who I was.

"Clint, this is my last day. I'm having transplant surgery tomorrow. I wanted to say goodbye."

Clint opened his eyes a little more.

"Okay, Miss D," he said, seeming still half asleep. "Good luck to you now. I mean that."

"Thank you, Clint," I said. "I know you do. Take care of yourself."

As I walked out the door, I wasn't sure if Clint had heard my last words or if he had gone back to sleep.

I must admit to feeling disappointed as I left the Center. I thought people would be sorrier to see me go. But then it occurred to me that the folks at dialysis are used to seeing people come and go. I also had a moment of real talk with myself as I made my way to the garage.

Girl, you ain't special! Besides, you were the one who didn't want to speak to any of those people not too long ago. Now you want them to be sorry to see you go?

My feelings of melancholy quickly disappeared when I saw Herbert, the parking lot attendant, wave to me signaling that he was going to get my car. When he pulled up and opened the door for me, I said, "Herbert, I'm going to miss you. You've been so kind to me. If I'm fortunate this will my last day at dialysis. I'm having a transplant tomorrow." I could hear myself almost singing those last five words.

Herbert stepped out of my car with a big grin on his face.

"Wow! Congrats Miss. Watson, I'll miss you too but I'm so glad to hear that. Good luck to you."

"Please give me a number where I can reach you. I'd like to stay in touch," I said to Herbert, as I folded an extra-large tip into his hand.

Herbert scribbled a number down on a torn piece of paper and handed it to me as we said goodbye. I later called the number a few times, but no one ever answered.

That night, Joe's son Hakimu spent the night at our house so he could drive us to the hospital. We arrived at Johns Hopkins at exactly 5:30 that Tuesday morning.

The attendants took Joe to the operating room first, although one of them had to pry our hands apart to roll his bed away. Afterward, the anesthetist came in to give me my first dose of medication. I lay in the bed alone behind a drawn white curtain for what seemed like a long time thinking about the last five years of my life—the pain, the blood, the vomit and urine, T, in the red Obama baseball cap I gave him. But I was fast losing touch with reality. I felt so tired. All I wanted was the sleep I knew was coming and the healthy, normal life I hoped was waiting for me on the other side.

Chapter Fifteen:
LOSS, LOVE, LIFE

One October morning about a month after my transplant, I opened my email to see a note with From Your Donor in the subject line. My hand froze. I wasn't certain I wanted to open the mail. Why are you hesitating, I thought to myself. You started this.

By "this" I meant that I'd started the communication between me and my "altruistic" kidney donor. The staff at Hopkins had been clear that in most transplants like mine, where the donor doesn't specify the recipient of their kidney, both parties remain anonymous. I heard more than once, "We have procedures in place to protect the anonymity of both patients."

However, on the morning I was to be discharged from the hospital, I felt a strong urge to thank this stranger for their priceless gift. Part of my feeling was a result of my upbringing. Growing up in my family, saying thank you for a nicety, no matter how large or small, was a must. Also, I was being discharged on a Monday and felt immensely grateful to be going home with a new, human kidney instead of to dialysis to be hooked up to a mechanical one.

"Would it be all right for me to leave a note for my donor?" I asked the transplant coordinator when she came around to say goodbye. "Regardless of how things are usually done, I'd like to thank them. You don't have to give me their name, but could you make sure that they get my note?"

The coordinator looked at me with what seemed like a mix of admiration and surprise.

"Sure, I can do that," she said. "Your donor will come in for a follow-up appointment at some point, or we can put it in the mail."

I don't remember the paper I used to write the note or even my exact words. I'm sure I graciously thanked this mysterious altruist for giving me another chance at a healthy life. Since I had no reason to stay anonymous, I included my name and contact information, inviting my donor to get in touch if they so desired. After a month passed and I didn't receive a response, I assumed that this person had never received my note, or even more likely, I thought, had chosen not to contact me.

Frankly, both possibilities were okay with me by then. While I still felt incredible gratitude toward this stranger, I was much more wrapped up in the recovery Joe and I were enjoying. We'd spent the weeks after surgery in a world of our own, waking up at our leisure, spending mornings watching reruns of the *The Sopranos*, and afternoons taking slow, careful walks around our neighborhood. According to the doctors, daily walks after surgery would speed the healing process and aid the return of normal bowel function. So, we walked, hand in hand, as in love as ever, and proud of what we'd overcome in our young marriage.

However, no matter how happy and content I was on that October morning, the unexpected response from "your donor" the person whose kidney I could feel in my body, jarred me. Who could she or he be? Did I want to know them? What was their story? I pressed the mouse. The note read in part, "You probably got the same prickles all over when you read this subject line as I did when I opened your note to me today. It was a shock to see your name and contact information. But now that you have identified yourself, I will identify myself as well.... I am a fifty-nine-year-old mom, wife and working woman (I work at USAID after a long career in US business). That kidney of yours has been many many places in the past few years due to my work—from Mali to Jakarta, Cambodia to Mexico, Peru to Kosovo, Rwanda to Bangladesh, and on and on. I'll stop now and let you absorb all this.... Respond if you wish but not if you do not want to do so." Judy Payne.

But I did want to respond. After reading her note, I was curious about "Judy," this world traveler who was a year older than me, shared a name with one of my sisters, and had voluntarily given up a body organ to someone she didn't know.

My donor, Judy, and I began an email correspondence which, because of her travel schedule, lasted months before we ever met in person. I told her about Joe and our sons, the rest of my family including my new granddaughter, my yoga practice, and my career as a non-profit executive, social policy writer, and consultant. She told me about her two daughters, her penchant for running and hiking, her husband, "a very nice guy," who worked for the World Bank, and more about the USAID work she loved. Judy helped farmers, small businesses, and other organizations in developing countries use technology to increase the success of development projects. I liked what I read about her.

Eventually, Judy and I exchanged pictures and learned about each other's races. I'd guessed that she was White after she told me she lived in McLean, Virginia, one of the most affluent communities in Virginia and the country. Intrigued, I asked her why she decided to donate her kidney to a stranger. I was flabbergasted by her email response, which read, "One day in early 2009 while looking at the news, I saw that a woman had donated one of her kidneys to former Mayor of DC Marion Barry so that he could have a transplant. Barry had suffered kidney failure in 2008 and was on dialysis. When I saw a picture of him and his donor together looking so happy, I thought, I can do that. I'm strong and healthy. My family was not in favor of me donating my kidney. My husband never said no but he didn't say yes either. My daughter, a doctor, said that if I insisted on donating, I should have the surgery at Hopkins since they were the best."

What amazed me about Judy's response was that Marion Barry was quite a racially polarizing figure who'd been arrested and convicted on drug charges in 2004 while serving as Mayor of the District. Who was this White woman who was motivated to altruism by Marion Barry's medical misfortunes?

Judy and I finally met in March 2010 at Mark's Kitchen, a neighborhood restaurant in Takoma Park, Maryland, the day after she returned from a work trip to Ethiopia. She looked exactly like her picture—a few inches taller than me with a thin, but athletic build, and short brown hair flecked with gray. Before our meeting, I'd been concerned about how I might feel in the presence of my donor. Would I feel pressure to express even more gratitude to Judy for her "gift"? Would she give off even the slightest whiff of superiority because she was White, or privileged (as she readily admits), or because she was the "donor"?

But after an hour or so of conversation, I felt none of those things. At the end of our meeting, when Judy looked at me earnestly and said, "I'd like to be friends," I shook my head in the affirmative. We continued to stay in touch through email, handwritten notes, family pictures, and occasional meals in restaurants and in each other's homes.

About a year after our first meeting, Judy and I sat again in Mark's Kitchen over tea, while she confided to me that, after more than thirty years of marriage, she and her husband were separating. A divorce was likely to follow. Judy did not want the divorce and confessed that she was "devastated."

"People in my family don't get divorced," she said glumly.

I touched Judy's hand. What could I say to my new friend that would make any difference in her sadness at this point? I wanted to try and remember saying something like these words, "Judy, who knows what life will bring? I don't know what it feels like to end a marriage of thirty-six years, but I've been through two divorces, and know that pain. I also know the strength it takes to pull yourself together and go on after a major loss. You have that strength, Judy. I've seen it. Now use it to take care of yourself."

I know my words weren't the only thing that motivated my donor Judy to get through her divorce and move on with her life. But I was happy to "gift" her a piece of advice from my own life. I hoped my words would be helpful in hers.

I remember having a definite spring in my step as I left Judy to walk home that day. I'd also walked from my house to our meeting in Takoma Park. *Good for you, ol' girl*, I thought to myself. Two miles round trip. Since my recovery, I'd been working toward resuming a life-long practice of walking several miles a week. I felt good. I believe that as I walked home, I started to hum a spiritual we used to sing in Tindley Temple, my childhood church. *I Don't Feel No Ways Tired.*

I was proud of my two-mile walk that day. But even more

than the pride I felt about walking, I felt grateful for the distance I'd traveled during my decades-long battle with the dreaded FSGS. In fact, over the years, gratitude had become a kind of religion for me—a saving grace. Of course, I was grateful for my donor Judy and her improbably compatible kidney. But I'd also received many other gifts along the way, some of which I didn't immediately appreciate.

As I walked home, I thought about my "imperfect" upbringing. There was no question that I'd emerged from my family wounded. But thankfully, through time, therapy, and struggle, I'd learned to acknowledge the pride, toughness, and discipline my parents had instilled in me. These qualities had served me well as I'd battled for my life. And despite our often distant, erratic relationship, my siblings, especially my sister Baby Alice, my first kidney donor, showed me that despite conflict, true family love ran deep.

I also thought of the patients I'd been in dialysis with at Fresenius Dialysis Center. Three in particular—Clint, T, and Cassandra, thankfully befriended me despite my initial unfriendliness. I cringed inside as I recalled how I judged and avoided the other patients, "those people," barely acknowledging them. However, dialysis treatment is a great "equalizer." One day during treatment, I was stripped of all pretentiousness when I vomited all over myself and was reduced to screaming and crying for a technician's help. I'd watch with aversion as other patients had suffered the same fate. On that day, I knew I'd been wrong. Despite my middle-class status, I was just as Black, sick, and vulnerable as everyone else in the room. "Those" people were "my people." I'll never forget them.

As the sun shined on the sidewalk, I thought about Robert, the only child I'd given birth to. I could almost see his shadow on the ground beside me. We used to walk everywhere together. Although I'd tried to shield him from the worst of my illness, I'd carried Robert in my heart through everything. He'd given me something to live for.

My steps quickened as I neared our house until I was practically running up the front steps, hoping Joe would be standing in the doorway. This is the "normal" life I've been craving, I thought. Was everything perfect? No. I knew the specter of FSGS would hang over me for the rest of my days. There was no cure, only pills designed to help me hold on to my new kidney. If I wanted to make it, I'd still have to be that tough South Philly girl. That's who I am at heart anyway.

And then there was Joe—the man I'd had sense enough to open my heart to; the man who'd already proven that he'd be by my side in sickness and in health. Was it gratitude I felt as I pushed open the door? Yes. I was home.

Epilogue:
FALL 2022

On Thursday, September 22, 2022, I celebrated thirteen years with my second transplanted kidney. In years past on this anniversary, my husband Joe and I would drive to Baltimore for a meal of pasta and garlic bread at Sabatino's, the Italian restaurant we frequented when we were preparing for transplant surgery back in 2009. This time the day came and went without either of us remembering its significance. When I recalled the anniversary a few days later, I dashed a "thinking of you today" note off to my donor, Judy, who now lives in New Hampshire. I also reminded Joe of the day.

"Did you remember that this past Thursday was the thirteenth anniversary of our kidney transplant surgery?" I asked Joe, somewhat smugly.

"Wow, I totally forgot," Joe responded. "Thirteen years! Want to drive up to Sabatino's and celebrate?"

I thought about Joe's suggestion for a moment but decided no. I was in for the day.

"I don't feel like going out, babe," I said. Let's just stay in and be grateful— count our blessings. We can always go up to Sabatino's another time."

I'm not sure if my forgetting the anniversary of our transplant surgery was a good or bad thing. On the one hand, I never want to take my successful transplant experience for granted. On the other hand, I think it's a good sign that my kidney surgeries aren't the most prominent things on my mind and that my transplanted kidney of thirteen years is working.

I can't forget that I've had two transplants even if I want to. My medicine case full of immuno-suppression, blood pressure, antibiotics, and other medications sits prominently on my kitchen counter. Doctors' appointments, most of them related to my transplant, dot my calendar. The pills and appointments remind me of the sobering truth that I'll be under medical supervision for the rest of my life.

Thankfully, my new kidney and I have done well together. Since my second transplant thirteen years ago, I've been in reasonably good health. I'm convinced that my ongoing yoga and meditation practices have been as beneficial as medication and excellent health care to my overall well-being. Admittedly, there have been a few scares. Twice, I've landed in the hospital because of medication interactions. And because my immune system is compromised, a few "bugs," including COVID, have laid me low for days on end. Of course, like many other transplant patients, I live with the side effects of immunosuppression medications such as puffiness, gastrointestinal issues, occasional tremors, and anxiety. But the bottom line is—I'm here.

A lot has happened in my life, in the country, and in the world over the past thirteen years. I'm not at all happy about the state of the country and world right now, with racial animus, political and economic turmoil, and war all raging. But for the most part, I'm grateful for the way things have progressed in my own life.

BERNARDINE WATSON

∼

By 2010, I'd recovered enough from my second transplant to begin thinking about what I wanted to do with the rest of my life. Initially, I planned to look for a full-time job in the leadership of a respectable nonprofit, or at least continue my consulting practice writing on social policy issues. DC seemed like fertile ground for those ambitions. I'd been an executive vice president at Public/Private Ventures, one of the most respected youth policy groups in the country, run my own consulting practice for several years and still had a contract with the Stoneleigh Foundation in Philadelphia. My husband, Joe, encouraged me in this direction. Joe has always been my biggest booster, encouraging me to take full advantage of my professional skills and talents.

I soon found job hunting tiresome, boring, and fruitless. After a year or so, I began to acknowledge a few truths. First, except for a few small contracts, I'd been out of the social policy market for four-to-five years. Second, during the years I was on dialysis and recovering from my kidney transplant, many of the contacts I'd built in the social policy world had moved on to other positions or left the field entirely. Some had been pushed out by the Great Recession of 2008, others by companies' desires to hire younger or less expensive staff. Third, I was sixty years old and likely experiencing age discrimination in the job market. Even further, I was in DC, a town where I had few contacts and where the competition is brutal. Even my lauded work on the important Pre-K for all DC project did not help me find work in the rough and tumble DC educational and political spheres.

Frankly, the more I hunted for a job or substantial consulting contract, the more I realized that I didn't truly want either. I wasn't sure exactly what I wanted in my future, but something fundamental had changed inside me. I no longer wanted a traditional, full-time job or demanding consulting assignment. If possible, I wanted and needed something where I could set my own pace, make my own choices, take care of my mental and physical health, and satisfy my soul. After so many years of hustling to earn a living, raising my son, and on top of all that, battling kidney disease, I wasn't even sure if what I was seeking was possible.

Joe certainly wanted me to be happy, but he didn't agree with my outlook right away.

"You know you're qualified to do any job out there," he said. "You also know how to take good care of yourself. Give it time. You'll find something worthy of your skills."

I looked at Joe deeply to see if I could detect anything besides the words he'd spoken. Then I asked him the question on my mind.

"Are you concerned about money, Joe? Are you concerned that you'll be the main breadwinner in our household? I know it's been that way while I've been sick. Are you looking forward to me going back to work full-time so we can have more money? I'll be able to officially retire soon, and I have my own savings."

I had to ask the question and, to this day, I appreciate Joe's honest answer.

"Baby, I won't lie. More money would be great, and you can command a good salary. But we're far from starving. I'll support whatever you decide to do."

Once Joe spoke on the subject, I had to get real with myself. How did I feel about being supported financially by my husband for who knows how long? After everything we'd been through, had I truly learned to accept his unconditional love and support? No matter what had happened in my life, I was still the same independent girl. Finally, I told myself that everything would be okay. I decided once again, to trust my husband, trust myself, and go ahead and live my life.

    I drifted for a while, looking for the best ways to balance care for my physical and mental health with "work" that felt satisfying and purposeful. Since writing has always been my basic skill, I knew that the written word would have a place in whatever I decided to undertake. I continued my work with the Stoneleigh Foundation for a while, writing a well-received series about their fellowship projects. I also freelanced for *The Washington Post*'s "She the People" blog, writing about juvenile justice, the civil rights movement, youth homelessness, and other social issues.

    In 2012, while out wandering around my neighborhood, I saw a flyer for a poetry workshop called "Writing the Body," designed for those who had experience with life-threatening or chronic illness. The name and purpose of the workshop touched me. I'd dabbled in poetry through the years and thought the workshop would allow me to revisit the form and express some of the feelings I had about my illness. What I didn't know at the time was that "Writing the Body" would change my life. Interestingly, I didn't immediately write poems about my specific experiences with FSGS, dialysis, or transplants. Instead, poetry writing opened me to telling the many other stories and feelings stored in my body. I wrote about my family, the South Philly neighborhood I grew up in, my friendships, police violence against Black people, and how it felt to be me, a Black woman, trying to survive and thrive in this country and world. Today, I still study with Anne Becker, the leader of the workshop. Although I haven't written many poems about my illness, the very act of writing poetry has been part of my healing and has become

TRANSPLANT: A MEMOIR

an essential part of my life. My poems have been published in numerous journals and anthologies and I've read my work in libraries, art and community centers, houses of worship, backyards, and on street corners across the DMV and Philadelphia. Poems about my time in the big blue chair are coming.

∽

UNFORTUNATELY, there are still no treatments for kidney failure, besides transplant and dialysis, although I now see ads on television for medicines designed to reduce the risk of further deterioration in diseased kidneys. The situation is so critical because, according to the National Institutes of Health, the incidence of kidney failure and FSGS is continuing to rise in the United States and the world. After my second transplant, I vowed to do what I could to share my story with others who might benefit. Frankly, I couldn't help anyone else until I was free of the rage and shame I felt about my kidney failure and being on dialysis.

I've volunteered with various organizations such as the National Kidney Foundation, NephCure Kidney International, American Association of Tissue Banks, National Institutes of Health, and Johns Hopkins Hospital. Speaking from my experience, I remind health providers to be sensitive to their patients and try to understand the fear, uncertainty, and stress that come with kidney failure, dialysis, or transplantation. I talk with patients and their families about how I learned to prioritize my physical and mental health, ask for help and support when I need it, and advocate for myself in the healthcare system. My two closest comrades in this battle, Joe, and my donor Judy Payne have participated in these forums with me. I hope their healthy presence alone encouraged others to consider kidney donation. In 2015, I wrote an article about my battle with kidney disease for *The Washington Post* Health and Science section titled, "Kidney Disease? But I Was Only 33 Years Old and Felt Fine." The piece ran with two large pictures of me. Thankfully, I am no longer afraid of people knowing about my health struggles.

I've also kept a promise to myself that I made back in 2006 when I was still deep in the belly of the beast. Back then, I vowed that when my head was clearer, I'd look more deeply into the discrepancies in kidney transplantation between African Americans and White people.

According to a 2017 article in the *American Journal of Nephology* titled "Health Disparities in Kidney Transplantation for African Americans," these disparities are still primarily unchanged, for many of the reasons I read about more than a decade ago, including limited kidney donors suitable for African Americans, inadequate access to care, low socioeconomic status and mistrust of clinicians and the healthcare system generally. Further, according to the National Kidney Foundation, Black patients face barriers to receiving a transplant at every step of the process and on average wait a year longer than White patients for the surgery. Black patients are less likely to receive a transplant evaluation, have less access to the waitlist, spend longer on the transplant waitlist, are less likely to survive on the waitlist, and have higher rates of losing their new kidney after the transplant.

While I was fortunate enough to access the kidney transplant system and have two successful transplants, I'm a witness to the reality that many of the resources available to me—excellent health insurance and medical care, financial security, willing donors, a husband who came through for me when I needed him most, and my own ability to navigate the health care system—are not available to many others.

Currently, I see some attempts at addressing racial disparities in kidney transplantation. Many of the forums that I've participated in with researchers, health providers, patients, and their families have been frank discussions about how to improve transplant outcomes for African Americans. I'm also aware of some potential systemic changes. The National Kidney Foundation is working with sponsors of the HealthEquity Accountability Act (HR 7585) to include provisions that focus on eliminating disparities in access to transplantation. If passed, the act could authorize programs that expand access to transplant education and counseling for Black and other communities of color and create a grant program providing monetary assistance to support low-income transplant candidates. Also, in June 2022, The Board of Directors of the Organ Procurement and Transplantation Network, the transplant system in the US, approved a measure to require transplant hospitals to use a "race-neutral" formula when determining eligibility for a kidney transplant.

And even more change is pledged. In March 2023, the Federal Health Resources and Services Administration announced an overhaul of the US organ transplant system itself. According to a March 22, 2023, article in *The Washington Post*, the system has long been criticized for long waiting lists for organs, most of them kidneys, "with poor and minority patients generally fairing worse than affluent and White people." *The Post* article states that early reaction on Capitol Hill appears positive on both sides of the isle and that patient advocates have also lauded the proposed overhaul.

Of course, these actions are welcome. However, so much more is needed to reduce kidney failure and the need for dialysis in the first place. Organizations such as the National Kidney Foundation (NKF) and NephCure Kidney International are working to increase public awareness of kidney disease so people can avoid kidney failure. Promising research into the early detection and treatment of FSGS, as well as other kidney diseases, is also underway. The pioneering work of Dr. Jeffrey Kopp at the National Institutes of Health, who I interviewed for a 2015 *Washington Post* article, has helped identify a gene variant found largely in West Africa which has been determined to be a powerful contributor to the risk of FSGS among African Americans. Study of this variant is ongoing at NIH, Mayo Clinic, and other medical research centers to determine its role in the development and progression of FSGS. This work is particularly interesting to me since when diagnosed with FSGS, I had none of the risk factors—heart disease, diabetes, obesity, or high blood pressure—except being of West African descent.

Black people have the highest rates in the country of high blood pressure, diabetes, obesity, and heart disease—the main risk factors for kidney disease. It follows that we are three times as likely as White people to suffer kidney failure and wind up on dialysis. Only recently, I learned that two of my first cousins suffered renal failure due to uncontrolled high blood pressure. Both spent time on dialysis—one died, the other was fortunate enough to receive a transplant.

A 2020 paper from researchers at John Hopkins Center for Health Equity lays out in breathtaking detail the role of race on kidney health in the Black Community. The paper titled, "Racial Disparities in Kidney Disease Contribute to Suffering and Premature Death for Black People," comes closer to anything else I've read, to reinforcing what I saw during my five years in a dialysis center. The study notes that Black people in this country are not predisposed to poor health. In fact, we are affected by racial discrimination in opportunities for housing, education, food, health care, and employment that contribute to these disparate outcomes. The study also expands on specific byproducts of racial discrimination such as exposure to repeated violence; living in food deserts where healthy food needed for preventing diabetes and heart disease is limited, and the lack of timely access to health care—which often means not being diagnosed until the disease is harder to treat or the kidneys have already failed.

The study also discusses the relationship between kidney disease and the concept of "weathering." The researchers define weathering as "eroded health caused by the repeated harmful experience of racism" and conclude that "the associated chronic stress caused by weathering, starts in the uterus and has a cumulative effect on mental and physical health throughout a lifetime." In other words, many African Americans end up with kidney failure or in a dialysis chair because they have had to "weather" the experience of being Black in America. The study even cites the COVID-19 epidemic as another adverse experience for Black kidney patients to "weather," since procedures like the insertion of access tubes and dialysis treatments create an added level of risk. Throughout the height of the pandemic, and still today, I think of people on dialysis and whisper words of gratitude for my transplant.

So, what's to be done to improve health outcomes for Black people facing kidney and other chronic diseases? The authors of this study say that "addressing the root causes of systemic racism" is the only answer. They suggest that: clinicians "see" and consider the myriad issues their Black patients are weathering; public health officials not just document structural problems in the health system but help develop solutions; and that each of us uses our platforms to advocate for meeting the basic needs of people of color and low income. I hope my book will contribute.

BERNARDINE WATSON

∼

SOMETIMES MEMORIES of Dupont Circle Dialysis Center—the blood, the needles, the cramps, the death, and the people I met there—haunt me. For years, after my last dialysis treatment, I passed by 11 Dupont Circle and promised myself that I would go in and visit with the staff and patients. But I never stopped. Then one Monday morning, about five years ago when I was in the area for another appointment, I did. My feet just seemed to walk in the direction of the building—past the Starbucks where I'd fainted after my first treatment in 2004, across New Hampshire Avenue, and into the building's courtyard. When I pulled the structure's heavy glass door open and headed for the elevator, the security guard looked up at me briefly, then went back to reading his paper. I pushed the button that pointed down.

I'm not sure what I expected when I walked into the Center at 10:00 on a Monday, which was during the time of my old treatment schedule. What I experienced was surreal. Someone wrapped tightly in a blanket was fast asleep in what was, for almost five years, my blue chair. The other sights, sounds, and smells of the place were all the same and came rushing back to overwhelm me. As I stood there, one of the staff began to walk toward me. I remembered him at once, because he'd been very kind to me when I was at the Center. His name was B.J. but I couldn't remember his title. I was surprised but glad that he recognized me too.

"Ms. Watson," he said. "How are you? You look great."

I stunned myself by throwing my arms around him and dissolving into tears. All I could say was "Thank you for taking care of me."

B.J. just patted me on the back and nodded as if my outburst was normal.

"You're well?" he asked standing back, taking a good look at me, and nodding yes himself as if he'd already decided that his assumption about my health was correct.

"Yes," I answered, before I began asking about "my people" one by one, hoping he would remember them as he remembered me.

"Is Nurse Margaret still here?"

B.J. shook his head, no. "She left a few years ago."

"David?" the handsome Jamaican and my favorite tech.

"He's working another shift and will be in later."

"Cammie?"

"Yes, Cammie Johnson," he responded. "I remember her. She had a transplant a few years ago."

Hallelujah! I thought. The young lady I couldn't help back then had found a way to help herself.

Finally, I summoned the nerve to ask about the people I most wanted to know about. "Did Mr. Wooley ever come back?" B.J. cocked his head to the side and looked as if he was trying to remember T, then shook his head no.

"I remember Mr. Wooley, but I don't know what happened to him."

At that moment, I could see T clear as day, leaning to one side and sporting the red Obama hat I'd given him.

"Clint? You remember Clint, right? He sat right over there." I pointed to Clint's old chair, which was empty, and could almost hear him calling out "hey, Miss D" as I walked by.

"Clint died a while ago," B.J. said. "He'd been here a long time."

Finally, I asked, "Where's Cassandra? She sat right next to me." Forgetting my mother's admonition not to point at people, I pointed to a chair where another woman was now sitting watching television.

B.J. sighed and looked down at the floor while I braced myself for the news.

"Cassandra died a few years ago. She had a sudden heart attack."

I couldn't speak for a moment. Beautiful Cassandra, who'd schooled me about how to stay warm during treatments; who'd struggled to care for her ailing father while she suffered with kidney disease and dialysis herself; who seemed beloved by the other patients. Cassandra, who never looked like she'd been sick one day in her life.

∾

I WILL TURN seventy-two years old on July 16 of 2023. Doctors have told me that the average life expectancy of a transplanted kidney is twenty-five years. If I'm average, I have seven to twelve years before my precious kidney gives out. But I've never thought of myself as average. According to research being conducted at The Ohio State University Wexner Medical Center, the longest a kidney transplant has lasted is sixty years. My first cousin, Ira, who I recently learned had a kidney transplant, has had his organ for twenty-four years.

I have no idea what the future will bring. In my daily meditations, I see myself as able to handle whatever comes. I'm still a tough South Philly girl. But truth be told, I want to continue, for as long as I can, living the lessons of trust, hope, gratitude, and generosity of spirit that I've learned in my battle with kidney disease. Of course, I'm also looking forward to many, many more nights of sacred sanctuary, on Fridays or otherwise, with my love, Joe.

BOOK CLUB DISCUSSION GUIDE

1. How would you react to a diagnosis of a deadly disease? Would your reactions be like Dine's or different?

2. In this memoir, the author reveals many intimate details about herself, including her illness, body, and relationships. She could have fictionalized this story. Why do you think she chose the memoir genre?

3. Reflect on Dine's relationship with her family, particularly with her father and her sister, Baby Alice. Do you empathize with her feelings about her family and her place in it? Why or why not?

4. Does the culture of secrecy that Dine describes in her family and community resonate with you? How do you think this culture shaped her reaction to her diagnosis?

5. Dine's friendships with those at the dialysis center took some time to evolve, but they were eventually deep and meaningful. Why do you think T, Clint, and Cassandra became so important to her?

6. It's often said that Black people don't go to therapy. What did you think of Dine's seeking therapy at different points in her illness? How do you think therapy helped or did not help her?

7. How do you think the issues of race and class are handled in this book? How do you think these factors affected Dine's—and others' medical treatment?

8. What did you learn about the American healthcare system in this memoir? In particular, did it make you think differently about organ donation?

9. The author says that *Transplant* is a story of personal change and transformation. Do you agree? What changes did Dine make? What experiences during her illness most influenced these changes?

More from the Washington Writers' Publishing House

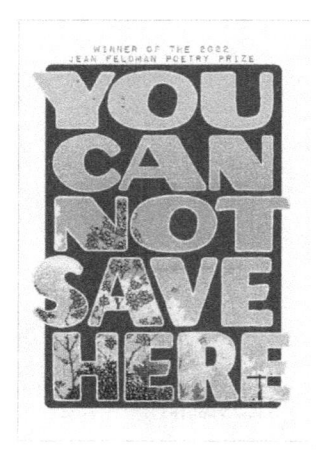

You Cannot Save Here
Tonee (Anthony) Moll

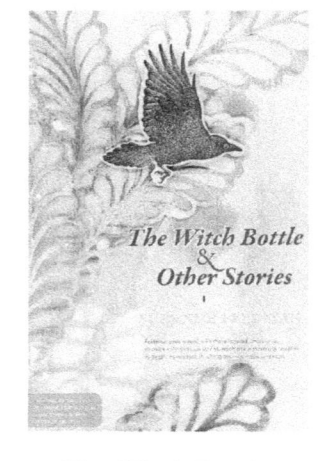

The Witch Bottle & Other Stories
Suzanne Feldman

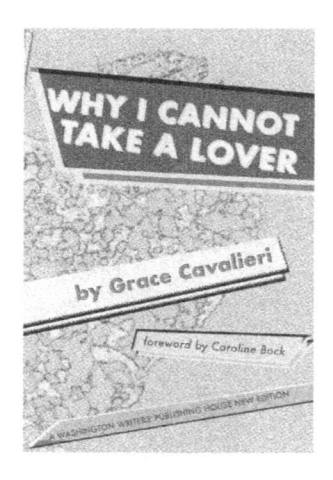

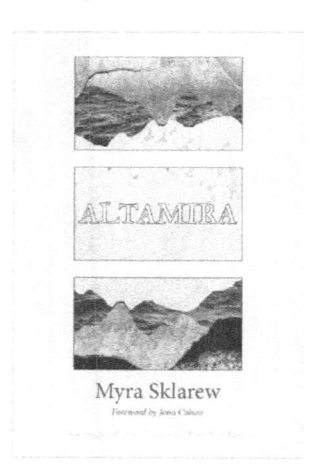

Why I Cannot Take a Lover
Grace Cavalieri

Altamira
Myra Sklarew

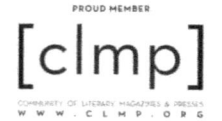

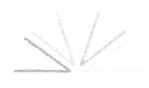

Washington Writers' Publishing House

Washington Writers' Publishing House (WWPH) is an independent, nonprofit, cooperative press founded in 1975. Our mission is to publish and celebrate writers from DC, Maryland, and Virginia. To learn more about our fiction, poetry, and creative nonfiction manuscript contests, our bi-weekly literary journal, *WWPH Writes*, and to purchase more WWPH books, please visit:

www.washingtonwriters.org

Follow us on:
Twitter: @wwphpress
Facebook: @WWPH
Instagram: @writingfromWWPH

Contact us at:
wwphpress@gmail.com

Sign up for our bi-weekly, online literary journal, *WWPH Writes*, by scanning the QR Code on the right. Free to subscribe and free to submit. Emails are only twice a month. Be part of the Washington Writers' Publishing House community, the (almost) 50-year-old cooperative, nonprofit literary press based in our nation's capital.